29/4/16

08 NOV 2016

Physical Medicine & Rehabilitation Pearls

TED A. LENNARD, MD

Clinical Assistant Professor
Department of Physical Medicine
University of Arkansas
Little Rock, Arkansas
 and
Private Practice
Springfield, Missouri

HANLEY & BELFUS, INC. / Philadelphia

Publisher: HANLEY & BELFUS, INC.
                    Medical Publishers
                    210 S. 13th Street
                    Philadelphia, PA 19107
                    (215) 546-7293, 800-962-1892
                    FAX (215) 790-9330
                    Website: http://www.hanleyandbelfus.com

Library of Congress Cataloging-in-Publication Data

Physical Medicine and Rehabilitation Pearls / edited by Ted A. Lennard.
       p. ; cm.—(The Pearls Series®)
    Includes bibliographical references and index.
    ISBN 1-56053-455-9 (alk. paper)
    1. Physical therapy—Case studies.   2. Medical rehabilitation—Case studies.
  I. Lennard, Ted A., 1961–   II. Series
    [DNLM: 1. Medicine—Case Report.   2. Medicine—Problems and Exercises.
  3. Rehabilitation—methods—Case Report.   4. Rehabilitation—methods—
  Problems and Exercises.   WB 18.2 P5778 2001]
  RM701.P4745 2001
  616'.09—dc21

                                                              00-069521

PHYSICAL MEDICINE AND REHABILITATION PEARLS   ISBN 1-56053-455-9

Last digit is the print number: 9 8 7 6 5 4 3 2 1

CONTENTS

Patient   **Page**

Patient **Page**

CONTRIBUTORS

Kenneth P. Botwin, MD
Fellowship Director, Florida Spine Institute, Clearwater, Florida

Martin K. Childers, DO
Associate Professor, Department of Physical Medicine and Rehabilitation, University of Missouri, Columbia; Rusk Rehabilitation Center, Columbia, Missouri

Jenness Doniphan Courtney III, MD
Northwest Louisiana Physical Medicine, Shreveport, Louisiana

Alice V. Fann, MD
Assistant Professor, Department of Physical Medicine and Rehabilitation, University of Arkansas for Medical Sciences, Little Rock; Central Arkansas Veterans Healthcare System, and University Hospital, Little Rock, Arkansas

Robert D. Gruber, DO
Medical Director, Florida Spine Institute, Clearwater, Florida

Navneet Gupta, MD
Chief Resident, Department of Physical Medicine and Rehabilitation, University of Arkansas for Medical Sciences, Little Rock, Arkansas

Florian S. Keplinger, MD
Assistant Professor, Department of Physical Medicine and Rehabilitation, University of Arkansas for Medical Sciences, Little Rock; Baptist Health Medical Center, and Little Rock Veterans Administration Medical Center, Little Rock, Arkansas

Thomas S. Kiser, MD, MPH
Assistant Professor, Department of Physical Medicine and Rehabilitation, University of Arkansas for Medical Sciences, Little Rock; University Hospital of Arkansas, and Baptist Health Rehabilitation Institute, Little Rock, Arkansas

Ashok Kumar, MD, FRCS
Clinical Assistant Professor, Division of Physical Medicine and Rehabilitation, Department of Neurology, Washington University School of Medicine, St. Louis, Missouri

Joshua D. Rittenberg, MD
Clinical Instructor, Department of Physical Medicine and Rehabilitation, Northwestern University Medical School, Chicago; Attending Physician, Rehabilitation Institute of Chicago, Chicago, Illinois

Stacy A. Rudnicki, MD
Associate Professor, Department of Neurology, University of Arkansas for Medical Sciences, Little Rock; University Hospital, Little Rock, Arkansas

Vikki Ann Stefans, MD, MS
Associate Professor, Departments of Pediatrics and Physical Medicine and Rehabilitation, University of Arkansas for Medical Sciences, Little Rock; Staff Physician and Medical Director of Progressive Rehabilitation Unit, Arkansas Children's Hospital, Little Rock, Arkansas

Santhosh A. Thomas, DO
Medical Director, Spine Center at the Cleveland Clinic Foundation, Westlake, Ohio

Francisco M. Torres, MD
Vice President, Florida Academy of Pain Management, Clearwater; Director of Osteoporosis Program, Florida Spine Institute, Clearwater, Florida

Andrew Michael Wayne, MD
Attending Physiatrist, Orthopedic and Sports Medicine, Inc., St. Louis; Clinical Instructor, Physical Medicine and Rehabilitation Residency Program, Washington University School of Medicine, St. Louis; Medical Director, Bridge Point Skilled Rehabilitation Center, St. Louis, Missouri

Jean You, MD
Resident, Department of Physical Medicine and Rehabilitation, University of Arkansas for Medical Sciences, Little Rock; University Hospital of Arkansas, and Baptist Health Rehabilitation Institute, Little Rock, Arkansas

PREFACE

This volume is a compilation of 85 diverse cases in physical medicine and rehabilitation. Many of these cases are complex and unique; others are simplistic and straightforward. All are thought provoking. The case studies are written to arouse curiosity, confirm clinical knowledge, and challenge diagnostic abilities.

The subjects of spinal cord injury, pain, stroke management, head injury, amputee management, and joint, spine, and neuromuscular diseases are addressed equally in this book. Both inpatient and outpatient rehabilitation issues are explored. There are select cases on commonly used drugs and drug pharmacology. Discussions on alternative medicine techniques for pain are also included. Each patient scenario was carefully chosen to represent a cross-section of our field, and the questions are designed to encourage you to think in new ways.

Each case is introduced with a succinct descriptive heading, followed by a short, pertinent historical perspective of the disease or injury process, physical examination findings, and, when appropriate, laboratory or radiologic data. Then, a question is posed to you. You will find the answer on the following page, as well as a discussion of the disease process, differential diagnosis, and injury or disease management. The discussion concludes with "take home" points called Clinical Pearls.

The authors' experiences are wide ranging, allowing expansive coverage of both the clinical and academic spectrum. All are experienced clinicians who have drawn from large patient populations. Many thanks go out to these authors for the invaluable time and effort they devoted to this book.

Enjoy!

Ted A. Lennard, MD
Editor

PATIENT 1

A 68-year-old man with diaphoresis and shortness of breath

A 68-year-old man became concerned when he experienced nausea, sweating, and malaise during a road trip. He had not eaten anything unusual, having packed his own meals and used fresh food. Later that same day, after returning home, the symptoms persisted with the addition of shortness of breath. He then went to the emergency room. He does not have fever, chills, or chest pain. History is significant for adult-onset diabetes (i.e., type II) of 10-year duration, in addition to peptic ulcer disease and hypertension.

Physical Examination: Temperature 98.2°, pulse 115, respirations 22, blood pressure 160/95. Skin: diaphoretic. HEENT: normal. Chest: clear. Cardiac: increased rate, regular rhythm, no murmurs. Abdomen: soft, nontender, normal bowel sounds. Costovertebral junction: nontender.

Laboratory Findings: WBC 6400/μl, Hct 39%, platelets 352,000/μl. Blood sugar 120 mg/dl. BUN 25 mg/dl, creatinine 1.2 mg/dl, trace glucose. Chest x-ray: lungs clear; heart mildly enlarged.

Question: What routine diagnostic study would have the highest yield in making the diagnosis?

Answer: Electrocardiogram (EKG)

Discussion: Coronary artery disease is the leading cause of morbidity and mortality in patients with diabetes. Diabetics have twice the morbidity and mortality related to myocardial infarction (MI) compared with nondiabetics. A **silent MI** is defined as a resting EKG-documented infarct in a person with either no classic symptoms of MI or atypical symptoms (nausea without chest pain). Diabetic patients often have MIs without classic chest pain because of their diminished sensory level. For that reason, other cardiac ischemia symptoms such as nausea, diaphoresis, and shortness of breath must be taken very seriously in a diabetic patient. This is especially true for **men with type II diabetes**, who have the highest prevalence of silent MI.

Regarding diagnosis, diabetic patients with suspected silent MI undergo the same work-up as nondiabetic patients: EKG, cardiac enzymes, chest x-ray, and cardiac angiogram and/or echocardiogram if indicated. The present patient's symptoms can also be seen in diabetic ketoacidosis; however, the essentially normal blood glucose level rules out that possibility.

Acute medical management includes oxygen and careful IV hydration, nitrates, thrombolysis, beta blockers, and angioplasty if needed. After the acute management, a **cardiac rehabilitation program** should be initiated. This program is divided into four phases: (1) The **acute phase** focuses on education and early mobilization, with continuous cardiac monitoring. (2) The **convalescent phase** continues with mobilization and moves toward increased endurance within the target heart rate determined at the end of the first phase. (3) The **training phase** starts with a symptom-limited exercise treadmill test to determine safe parameters for continued exercise. Cardiac monitoring is used less, and more emphasis is placed on patient self-monitoring. (4) The **maintenance phase** focuses on long-term exercises for muscles used in the earlier phases. Ideally, the exercises address muscles that are used in the patient's everyday vocational and avocational activities. The maintenance phase is meant to be a life-long routine.

The present patient will benefit from cardiac rehabilitation not only in terms of the cardiac effects and cardiac risk factor modification, but also in terms of diabetic control, including improved glucose metabolism and insulin sensitivity. In addition, cardiac rehabilitation has been shown to reduce depression and anxiety. This is especially important for diabetic patients because they have a significantly higher incidence of depression compared with their nondiabetic counterparts.

In the present patient, an EKG showed marked ST segment elevation in leads V1–V6 associated with early development of Q waves in leads V2 and V3 (*see figure*). This pattern usually reflects proximal occlusion of the left anterior descending artery (LAD). A cardiac catheterization revealed 70% stenosis in the LAD, 55% in the right coronary artery, and 52% in the circumflex branch. He was treated with tissue plasminogen activator for thrombolysis. An echocardiogram revealed mild left ventricular hypokinesis and an ejection fraction of 52%, but no valvular dysfunction. The cardiologist diagnosed a mild baseline diabetic cardiomyopathy with development of an acute MI in the left anterior ventricle. The findings on the cardiac catheterization are typical for a diabetic patient, because while there is no significant difference in the incidence of severe coronary artery stenosis between diabetic and nondiabetic patients, the diabetic patients have an increased incidence of *moderate* stenosis, which is more diffuse.

After his serial cardiac enzymes normalized, the patient initiated the acute phase of cardiac rehabilitation; subsequent phases were done outpatient, and he continued to exercise regularly. He was started on an ACE inhibitor during his hospitalization for better blood pressure control and to reduce the workload on his heart. He was already on a beta blocker, which was continued due to its effect on reducing the rate of MI reoccurence and sudden death. He was also started on a low cholesterol diet. His cardiologist stressed to him the importance of adhering to the lifestyle changes, and having more regularly scheduled medical follow-ups.

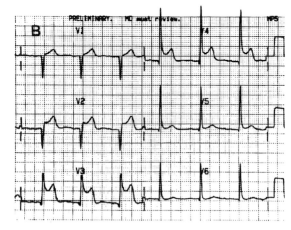

Clinical Pearls

1. Diabetic patients who are undergoing cardiac ischemia often present without angina.

2. While cardiac disease is the leading cause of morbidity and mortality in the U.S. adult population, diabetic patients experience twice the morbidity and mortality compared with nondiabetic patients.

3. Diabetic patients with MI have a lower baseline ejection fraction, reduced compensatory ability of the noninfarcted myocardium, and more extensive coronary artherosclerosis than their nondiabetic counterparts.

4. While there is no significant difference in the incidence of severe coronary artery stenosis between diabetic and nondiabetic patients, the diabetic patients have an increased incidence of *moderate* stenosis, which is more diffuse.

5. Psychological benefits of cardiac rehabilitation are especially vital for people with diabetes, due to their higher incidence of depression compared with nondiabetic patients.

6. The patient's EKG pattern usually reflects proximal occlusion of the LAD.

REFERENCES

1. Aronson D, Rayfield EJ, Chesebro JH: Mechanism determining course and outcome of diabetic patients who have had acute myocardial infarction. Ann Intern Med 126(4):296–306, 1997.
2. Henry P, Makowski S, Richard P, et al: Increased incidence of moderate stenosis among patients with diabetes: Substrate for myocardial infarction? Am Heart J 134(6):1037–1043,1997.
3. Janand-Delenne B, Savin B, Habib G, et al: Silent myocardial infarction in patients with diabetes: Who to screen. Diabetes Care; 22(9):1396–1400, 1999.
4. Lavie CJ, Milani RV: Benefits of cardiac rehabilitation and exercise training. Chest 117(1): 5–7, 2000.
5. Moldover JR, Bartels MN: Cardiac rehabilitation. In Braddom RL (ed): Physical Medicine and Rehabilitation. Philadelphia, WB Saunders Company, 1996, pp 649–670.
6. Nesto RW: Screening for asymptomatic coronary artery disease in diabetics. Diabetes Care 22(9): 1393–1395,1999.

PATIENT 2

A 32-year-old woman with a painful, extended right toe

A 32-year-old woman presents to a PM&R outpatient clinic with a 3-month history of pain in the right great toe. Past medical history is significant for a hemorrhagic stroke 6 months ago, with resulting right spastic hemiparesis. She has complained of toe pain ever since she began ambulating after her stroke. She notices pain along the top of the great toe with weight bearing. To accommodate this difficulty, the patient walks only with slippers, sandals, or canvas tennis shoes with a hole cut out over the great toe.

Physical Examination: Neurologic: reflexes brisk on right when compared to left; marked Babinski response on right; 4–5 beats of clonus elicited in right ankle; pulses brisk. Skin: dorsal surface of right great toe erythematous and tender to touch; nail bed unremarkable; color pink and without rashes. Musculoskeletal: no joint effusion or pain in any digits of right foot; motor power decreased by at least 1 grade (of 5) throughout muscles in right limb compared to left. Gait: slow and typical of spastic hemiparesis, and on affected right side during stance phase, patient is able to slowly rotate over ankle; however, striking abnormality present—great toe extends upward and remains extended when patient places weight on right foot (see figure).

Laboratory Findings: EMG of right lower limb: continuous motor unit firing (abnormal muscle contraction) of extensor hallicus longus on extension of right great toe; also when bottom of foot stroked, or when patient placed foot upon a surface.

Question: What procedure might be most effective in reducing pain in this condition?

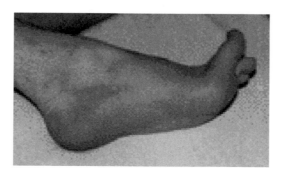

From Mayer NH, Esquenazi A, Childers MK: Common patterns of clinical motor dysfunction. Muscle Nerve 20 (suppl 6):S21–S35, 1997; with permission.

Answer: Botulinum toxin injection

Discussion: This condition is commonly termed "hitchhiker's toe" or "striatal toe" and is seen most often as the result of a stroke. More specifically, this condition results from **focal dystonia**, or inappropriate muscle contraction likely due to injury to the basal ganglia. While there is no specific confirmatory laboratory test to make such a diagnosis, EMG findings may be helpful to identify the specific muscle or muscles that are involved.

Botulinum toxin type A (BTX-A) has been reported to be effective in treating focal dystonias. (BTX-A is licensed for use in the United States for the treatment of blepharospasm, strabismus, and hemifacial spasm.) In this case, local injection of 50 units of BTX-A into the right extensor hallicus longus is recommended for focal dystonia resulting in hitchhiker's toe. Use EMG guidance—via a dual-purpose EMG recording needle with a port adapted for simultaneous injection—to carefully identify the abnormally contracting muscle.

In the present patient, 50 units of BTX-A was injected into the affected muscle clinically implicated as the cause of "striatal toe," the extensor hallicus longus (EHL) muscle. Three weeks following this treatment, the patient reported complete cessation of involuntary great toe extension, and decreased pain in the top of the great toe. The patient subsequently experienced continued relief of both involuntary muscle contraction of the EHL and pain in the great toe for a period of 4 months. Symptoms gradually returned, and subsequent injections of BTX-A brought about similar results, with the effects lasting 3–4 months.

Clinical Pearls

1. A diagnosis of "hitchhiker's toe" can often be made upon entering the examination room by observing the tell-tale sign of an opening cut in a tennis shoe over the great toe.

2. Proper needle entry into the extensor hallicus longus is sometimes difficult. Palpation over the expected muscle location while flexing and extending the great toe may be helpful in identifying the EHL muscle and tendon.

REFERENCES

1. Anonymous: Consensus conference. Clinical use of botulinum toxin. National Institutes of Health. [review] Conn Med 55:471–477, 1991.
2. Childers MK: Use of Botulinum Toxin Type A in Pain Management. New York, DEMOS Medical Publishing, 1999.
3. Markham CH: The dystonias. [review] Curr Opin Neurol Neurosurg 5(3):301–377, 1992.
4. Mayer NH, Esquenazi A, Childers MK: Common patterns of clinical motor dysfunction. Muscle Nerve suppl 6:21–35, 1997.

PATIENT 3

A 67-year-old woman with muscle cramps and weakness

A 67-year-old woman presents with muscle cramps and weakness of 1-year duration. She has been referred by her rheumatologist to the electrodiagnostic lab to confirm a tentative diagnosis of polymyositis. She was prescribed prednisone for her symptoms, but had noted no improvement. A muscle biopsy and an EMG have not been performed.

Physical Examination: Extremities: weakness both distally and proximally in arms and legs; wasting of intrinsic hand muscles (left more than right). Neurologic: diffusely brisk deep tendon reflexes; positive Babinski sign on left.

Laboratory Findings: See results of nerve conduction and EMG studies below.

Question: What do the study results demonstrate?

Nerve Conduction Study

Nerve	Site	Latency	NCV	Amplitude	F wave
R Median (m)	wrist-APB	4.5 ms		2.25 mV	29.1 ms
	elbow-wrist		51.5 m/s	1.92 mV	
R Ulnar (m)	wrist-ADM	2.6 ms		8.70 mV	31.2 ms
	below elb-wrist		51.4 m/s	7.0 mV	
	above elb-bel elb		56.8 m/s	7.40 mV	
R Tibial (m)	med mall-AH	5.2 ms		0.41 mV	
	knee-med mall		39.4 m/s	0.41 mV	
L Tibial (m)	med mall-AH	5.4 ms		0.22 mV	
	knee-med mall		41.8 m/s	0.22 mV	
R Median (s)	dig III-wrist	2.4 ms	50.8 m/s	24.20 μV	
R Ulnar (s)	palm-wrist	1.4 ms	57.0 m/s	10.0 μV	
R Median (s)	palm-wrist	1.6 ms	50.0 m/s	29.7 μV	
R Sural (s)	calf-lat mall		36.3 m/s	7.50 μV	

(m) = motor nerve, (s) = sensory nerve, NCV = nerve conduction velocity, APB = abductor pollicis brevis, ADM = abductor digiti minimi, AH = abductor hallucis, med mall = medial malleolus, lat mall = lateral malleolus

EMG Study

Muscle	Fibs	PSWs	Fascic	MUAP dur	MUAP amp	MUAP config	Int Pat
R Tib Ant	3+	3+	0	nl	inc	nl	red
R Med Gastr	1+	3+	0	occ inc	nl	occ pph	red
R Vast Lat	0	1+	1+	occ inc	nl	occ pph	red
R FDI	2+	2+	0	nl	large	nl	red
R EDC	2+	2+	0	nl	nl	nl	full
R Biceps Br	2+	2+	0	occ inc	nl	occ pph	full
L FDI	3+	3+	0	occ inc	nl	occ pph	red
L EDC	2+	2+	0	occ inc	nl	occ pph	red
L Biceps Br	1+	0	0	occ inc	nl	occ pph	full
L Cerv Parasp	1+	1+	0	occ inc	nl	pph	
R Cerv Parasp	2+	2+	0	occ inc	nl	pph	
R L-S Parasp	2+	2+	0	occ inc	nl	pph	

PSW = positive sharp waves, MUAP = motor unit action potential, Int Pat = interference pattern, FDI = first dorsal interosseous, EDC = extensor digitorum communis, inc = increased, nl = normal, pph = polyphasic, red = reduced

Diagnosis: Amyotrophic lateral sclerosis (ALS)

Discussion: The nerve conduction study reveals a preservation of sensory nerve action potential (SNAP) amplitudes with reduction of compound muscle action potential (CMAP) amplitudes. Overall, nerve conduction velocities (NCV) and distal latencies are normal. On EMG, findings are compatible with extensive acute denervation and chronic reinnervation in multiple muscles of the extremities and paraspinals. There has been a drop-out of motor units in many of her muscles, which resulted in a reduction of the interference pattern. This patient's profile—with a reduction of CMAP amplitudes and preserved SNAP amplitudes—is relatively uncommon in muscle disease. In general, the myopathies affect proximal muscles more than distal ones. Because routine nerve conductions studies evaluate only the distal muscles, changes on these studies are rare in myopathies.

In this patient, the EMG abnormalities are clearly due to a neurogenic etiology rather than a myopathic one. The clinical evaluation revealed evidence for **upper** *and* **lower motor neuron dysfunction**, thereby raising the suspicion of ALS. In many patients with ALS, nerve conduction studies may be completely within normal limits; however, CMAP amplitudes may be reduced and NCV may be mildly slowed. Sensory studies are normal, with rare exception. The EMG results typically show evidence of widespread acute denervation (including fibrillation potentials and positive sharp waves) and chronic reinnervation. Fasciculations, frequently apparent on visual inspection of the muscle, can also be seen electromyographically. Changes that are evidence of chronic reinnervation include motor unit action potentials with increased amplitude and polyphasic morphology. These changes are due to collateral sprouting of the remaining nerves. The interference pattern is decreased, and the remaining motor units fire at a faster frequency.

In confirming a diagnosis of ALS, **helpful hallmarks** such as EMG changes in three extremities with three muscles supplied by different nerve roots and nerves in each extremity give some substantiation. For these evaluations the head and neck may be considered an extremity. The examiner may also find abnormalities in the paraspinal muscles and the muscles of the tongue and face. Another commonly accepted electrophysiologic criteria for ALS requires that there be EMG changes in at least three of the following regions: brainstem, cervical, thoracic, or lumbosacral. Since the diagnosis of ALS requires examination evidence of upper motor neuron dysfunction along with lower motor neuron dysfunction, electrophysiology may *support* the diagnosis, but cannot itself *establish* the diagnosis.

Clinical Pearls

1. If sensory nerve conduction studies are normal, and motor nerve conduction studies reveal reduced amplitudes, then include motor neuron disease, Lambert-Eaton myasthenic syndrome, muscle disease, and pure motor neuropathy in the differential diagnosis.

2. On initial clinical presentation, ALS may mimic a number of other neurologic diseases. CPK can be elevated (up to 3 fold) in motor neuron disease and lead to the suspicion of a primary muscular disorder rather than ALS, further adding to the possibility of misdiagnosing the disease.

3. Clinically weak muscles should be evaluated first with needle EMG to assess for evidence of denervation and reinnervation. Even muscles that are normal in strength on clinical evaluation may demonstrate electrophysiologic changes.

4. Fasciculations can be present in normal muscle. These benign fasciculations are not associated with fibrillations, positive sharp waves, or motor unit potential changes.

REFERENCES
1. Criteria for the diagnosis of amyotrophic lateral sclerosis. A workshop entitled Clinical Limits of ALS. World Neurol 5:12, 1990.
2. Daube JR: Electrophysiologic studies in the diagnosis and prognosis of motor neuron disease. Neurol Clinics 3:473–493, 1985.
3. De Carvalho M, Swash M: Nerve conduction studies in amyotrophic lateral sclerosis. Muscle Nerve 23:344–352, 2000.
4. Denys EH: AAEM Case report #5: Amyotrophic lateral sclerosis. Muscle Nerve 17:263–268, 1994.
5. Rowland LP: Diagnosis of amyotrophic lateral sclerosis. J Neurol Sci 160S:S6–S24, 1998.

PATIENT 4

A 19-year-old man with traumatic brain injury and fever

A 19-year-old man sustained a traumatic brain injury in a head-on motor vehicular accident. Prolonged extrication by the emergency response team was documented. His initial Glasgow Coma Scale was 4 (eyes–2, motor–1, verbal–1). He was admitted and medically stabilized. After 10 days, he was transferred to the brain injury unit of a rehabilitation hospital. On the day of transfer, he was noted to have fever, diaphoresis, tachycardia, and hypertension, with intermittent decerebrate posturing. Medications include respiratory treatments with albuterol and saline updrafts, phenytoin 200 mg q 12 hours, famotidine 20 mg q 12 hours, ibuprofen 400 mg q 8 hours PRN, alternating with acetaminophen 500 mg q 8 hours, all administered through the gastrostomy tube.

Physical Examination: General: extensor posturing in all limbs in response to any stimulation, Rancho los Amigos level 2. Temperature 103.1°, pulse 120, respiration 28, blood pressure 170/80. Skin: cool and clammy, with profuse sweating. HEENT: tracheostomy connected to humidified air. Cardiac: tachycardic. Chest: clear. Abdomen: gastrostomy tube; soft; normal bowel sounds. Extremities: no edema or asymmetry.

Laboratory Findings: WBC 8500/μl, Hct 40%, platelets 274,00/μl. Urinalysis and urine culture: normal. Aerobic and anaerobic blood cultures: negative. Phenytoin level 14. Chest x-ray: see figure. Venous Dopplers: negative for deep venous thrombosis.

Question: What is the cause of this patient's fever?

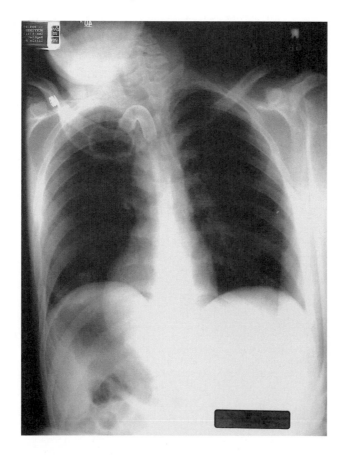

Diagnosis: Central fever associated with a hyperadrenergic state

Discussion: Post-traumatic fever can be caused by infection, atelectasis, aspiration without pneumonia, thrombophlebitis, and medications. All of these causes should be investigated before calling the fever of central origin.

In this patient, the physical exam, lab tests, and chest x-ray were normal. The tracheostomy tube was in place, and there was no evidence of pneumonia, pleural effusion, or atelectasia.

Central fever is often associated with other manifestations of the hyperadrenergic state: tachycardia, hypertension, and hyperhidrosis. These have been found to correlate with high elevations in plasma and urine catecholamine levels. The hyperadrenergic state is usually seen in severe traumatic brain injury.

Management consists initially of cooling blankets and attention to hydration. Useful medications include acetaminophen and nonsteroidal anti-inflammatory drugs, such as ibuprofen and indomethacin, for fever. Tachycardia and hypertension are preferably treated with beta-blockers (such as propranolol and atenolol), due to these drugs' effects on decreasing plasma catecholamines, thus decreasing heart rate and myocardial oxygen demand.

Initially, low doses should be used and then increased gradually, with monitoring of blood pressure and heart rate. Vasodilating agents should be avoided as they may increase cerebral perfusion pressure, putting the patient at risk of brain swelling. Centrally acting antihypertensive agents should likewise be avoided because of their sedating properties.

The present patient responded well to low-dose atenolol.

Clinical Pearls

1. Prolonged extrication and a low initial Glasgow Coma Scale score indicate not only traumatic, but also ischemic brain injury.

2. Perform a thorough investigation to rule out/in all possible causes of fever before attributing it to central origin.

3. Beta-blockers are preferred for post-traumatic hypertension associated with the hyperadrenergic state, since vasodilating agents can cause increased cerebral perfusion pressure, and centrally acting agents can cause sedation.

REFERENCE

Rosenthal M, Griffith ER, Kreutzer JS, Pentland B (eds): Rehabilitation of the Adult and Child with Traumatic Brain Injury, 3rd ed. Philadelphia, FA Davis Co, 1999.

PATIENT 5

A 9-year-old girl with unexplained cerebral palsy, microcephaly, and seizures

This 9-year-old girl has been followed in clinics since birth with a diagnosis of spastic quadriparetic cerebral palsy, but she is a new patient for you. You note a birth history of term delivery, birth weight 7 lbs even, and microcephaly. Seizures developed at 3 years of age and are reasonably controlled on Dilantin. She is non-verbal, walks with help, and attends special school, remaining dependent in most activities of daily living. Her family asks about the prognosis for talking and also wonders why she has this disability since no one else in the family is affected.

Physical Examination: General (see figure): weight 25th percentile, height 15th percentile, head circumference just under 5th percentile; she is drooling but alert, vocalizes some, and turns to sound. Spine: moderate S-curved scoliosis. Extremities: ataxic-like movements; some spasticity; unusual, tremorous, increased tone; marked valgus foot position without orthotics.

Laboratory Findings: Prior amino acid screens, thyroid studies, MRI of head: normal. Spine and hip x-rays: hips in place; curve maximally 30° in lower thoracic area with 27° compensatory curve above that. Chromosomal analysis (performed in 1993): 46 XX.

Questions: What condition does this child actually have? Which test needs to be performed or repeated?

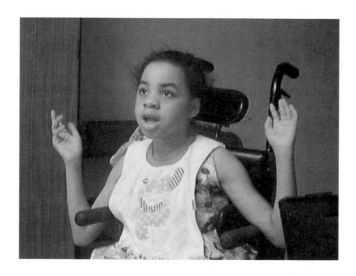

Diagnosis: Angelman syndrome. The confirmatory test is chromosome analysis with fluorescent in-situ hybridization for the specific chromosome involved, the 15q11-q13 region.

Discussion: When this chromosome is of maternal origin, the Angelman phenotype generally results; if paternal in origin, the child will have Prader-Willi syndrome. Exceptions occur with a less common condition of uniparental disomy, which can be either parent and still result in Angelman syndrome. Verbal speech is extraordinarily rare to nonexistent in this condition, but some children do use augmentative-alternative communication effectively, and it should be investigated. There is an active and helpful national support organization as well.* These children can also be mistakenly considered to have autism, but in fact this is not the case. Valgus feet are nearly universal and may be difficult to manage, sometimes requiring surgery.

In addition to Prader-Willi, several other genetic conditions may masquerade as cerebral palsy, such as Williams syndrome and Langer-Giedion syndrome. It is advisable to become familiar with them as this knowledge can be a great help to patients and their families.

Clinical Pearls

1. Children with unusual or unexplained features and conditions for which there is no explanation should be periodically reassessed with genetic testing.
2. "Cerebral palsy" in a term baby without explanation needs to be fully explored.
3. When working with families of "cerebral palsy" patients, realize that they react differently when receiving information about a new diagnosis. Offer the new information supportively, with ample opportunity for feedback, and provide referrals for more information.

* Angelman Syndrome Foundation, USA National Office
414 Plaza Drive, Suite 209
Westmont IL 60559
1-800-432-6435 (1-800-IF-ANGEL)
http://www.angelman.org

REFERENCES
1. Clarke DJ, Marston G: Problem behaviors associated with 15q- Angelman syndrome. Am J Ment Retard 105(1):25–31, 2000.
2. Fridman C, Varela MC, Kok F, Diament A, Koiffmann CP: Paternal UPD15: further genetic and clinical studies in four Angelman syndrome patients. J Med Genet 92(5):322–327, 2000.
3. Jones KL, Smith DW: Smith's Recognizable Patterns of Human Malformation. Philadelphia, W.B. Saunders Company, 1996.

PATIENT 6

An 82-year-old man with acute low back pain

An 82-year-old man presents with a 10-day history of low back pain which developed when unrolling a bale of wire while repairing a fence. At the time of injury the pain radiated into his left hip and anterior thigh, and he experienced numbness in the region of the anterior thigh. He also noticed discoloration in the proximal leg and groin. He initially treated himself with bedrest and aspirin, but sought the help of a chiropractor after 6 days with no pain relief. His back was treated with manipulation and adjustment, but his pain worsened. Eight days after the initial injury he was taken to the local emergency department by ambulance because his back pain was so severe. He was given ketorolac intravenously, resulting in some relief, and a follow-up 15-mg dose 2 hours later provided complete relief. He was discharged to home after 5 hours in the emergency department with the diagnosis of a muscular back strain, a prescription for Tylenol with codeine, and an appointment to see you. Now, he complains of fatigue and a weak and unstable left leg. He has started to use a cane.

Physical Examination: Pulse 160; respiration 18; temperature 97.8°; blood pressure 100/60. HEENT: normal. Chest: clear. Cardiac: tachycardiac and irregular. Extremities: normal bilateral pedal pulses. Abdomen: nontender with normal bowel sounds. Musculoskeletal: normal peripheral joints; back painful with any movement and mildly tender to palpation. Neurologic: left anterior thigh numb to touch and pinprick; normal muscle stretch reflexes; negative straight leg raising test; manual muscle test normal except for subtle hip weakness associated with back pain. Skin: ecchymoses of the left flank, gluteal, and thigh.

Laboratory Findings: Hct 21.1%; platelets 349,000/µl; prothrombin time 12.8 seconds; partial thromboplastin time 59 seconds; bleeding time 3.5 minutes (2.5-10); factor VIII assay < 3% (40–150%); factor IX assay 85% (40–150%); fibrin split products normal. ECG: premature ectopic complexes; otherwise normal. Abdominal ultrasound: normal aorta and proximal iliac vessels. CT scan: left pelvic hematoma displacing psoas muscle and iliac vessels. Aortic angiogram: smooth iliac vessels; no aneurysm or extravasation.

Question: What is the cause of this patient's back pain?

Diagnosis: Retroperitoneal hemorrhage secondary to acquired hemophilia.

Discussion: Retroperitoneal hemorrhage can mimic lumbar disc disease and cause low back pain. It presents as abdominal pain 60% of the time and back pain 25% of the time. **Grey Turner's** sign (ecchymosis of the flank) usually appears after a lapse of a few hours in a large bleed. As much as 2000–4000 cc can accumulate in the retroperitoneal space. Eighty percent of patients have hematuria, and a psoas shadow is obliterated in 30% of patients with anteroposterior x-ray of the spine.

Pelvic fractures are the most common traumatic cause of retroperitoneal hemorrhage. Nontraumatic causes are a leaking abdominal aortic aneurysm or dissection, duodenal perforation, hemorrhagic pancreatitis, ruptured ectopic pregnancy, and bleeding diatheses.

One of the most common causes of retroperitoneal hemorrhage in the elderly is a leaking aortic aneurysm or dissection. This was the initial working diagnosis in this case before the laboratory data was obtained. Acute aneurysmal rupture commonly occurs into the retroperitoneum on the left beneath the sigmoid colon, which can irritate the left lumbosacral plexus. Erosion of an aneurysm into the lumbar spine can cause symptoms of low pack pain. An abdominal aortic dissection usually is associated with a severe tearing pain as well as decreased pulses in the feet.

Acquired hemophilia is a rare condition, with a reported incidence of 1 in 1 million. It can arise spontaneously in association with a chronic inflammatory disease, pregnancy, or drug reactions. In the elderly it can occur in the absence of underlying disease. The pattern of bleeding differs from that of the congenital disorder in that hemarthroses are uncommon, and soft tissue bleeding is frequent. Hematuria and retroperitoneal hemorrhage are common in patients with acquired hemophilia.

The present patient had **factor VIII inhibitors**, which caused the acquired hemophilia. Treatment options are discussed in detail by Hoyer and by Green. Immunosuppression with corticosteroids and/or oral cyclophosphamide is the most common treatment. Coadministration of factor VIII with immunosuppression is sometimes attempted if inhibitors persist. Success with plasmapheresis, intravenous immunoglobulin, and protein A immunoabsorption has been reported. Spontaneous disappearance of the antibody has been described, particularly in pregnancy.

He was treated with oral coricosteroids. His factor VIII assay returned to normal, and the retroperitioneal hematoma and ecchymosis on his flank slowly resolved. His back pain also slowly resolved, and he was able to return to his normal active lifestyle.

Clinical Pearls

1. Acute low back pain is usually benign and self-limiting, but a treating physician must be alert for red flags, which may suggest more significant pathology.

2. Grey Turner's sign can appear within hours after a retroperitoneal bleed; therefore, conduct a thorough skin exam in a patient with acute low back pain, especially with a nontraumatic mechanism of injury.

3. There are many possible causes of retroperitoneal hemorrhage. If it is suspected, a systematic investigation is required. In this case, a simple laboratory test was the key to diagnostic success.

REFERENCES

1. Bithell TC: Acquired coagulation disorders. In Lee GR, et al (eds): Wintrobe's Clinical Hematology, 9th ed. Philadelphia, Lea & Febiger, 1993, pp 1473–1514.
2. Bonica JJ, Johansen K, Loeser JD: Abdominal pain caused by other diseases. In Bonica JJ (ed): The Management of Pain, 2nd ed. Philadelphia, Lea & Febiger, 1990, pp 1254–1282.
3. Green D: Immunosuppression of factor VIII inhibitors in nonhemophilic patients. Semin Hematol 30(suppl 1):28–31, 1993.
4. Green D, Lechner K: A survey of 215 nonhaemophilic patients with inhibitors to factor VIII. Thromb Haemost 45:200–203, 1981.
5. Hoyer LW: Hemophilia A. New Engl J Med 330:38–47, 1994.
6. Shires GT, Thal ER, Jones RC, et al: Trauma. In Schwartz SI (ed): Principles of Surgery, 6th ed. New York, McGraw-Hill, 1994, pp 175–224.

PATIENT 7

A 77-year-old woman with low back pain radiating into her lower extremities

A 77-year-old woman presents for evaluation of increasing low back pain, which radiates into the lower extremities. The pain is of 3-year duration. She has no history of recent trauma. She has a known history of hypertension, osteoporosis, hyperlipidemia, hypercholesterolemia, and peripheral arterial occlusive disease. Standing and walking as well as supine bed positioning aggravates her pain. She gets relief with sitting and home heating modalities. Her pain distribution is 10% lower back and 90% lower extremities. She denies numbness or tingling in the lower extremities. Her leg pain is greater in the right leg. She states that the pain radiates through the outer thigh into the front of her leg and down to the top of the foot.

Physical Examination: General: well developed, well nourished; no evidence of atrophy or fasciculation. Neurologic: non-antalgic gait; ability to heel and toe walk present; static and dynamic balance good; no gross sensory deficits to pin prick testing. Lumbar spine: no evidence of deformity, other than exaggeration of thoracic kyphosis. Musculoskeletal: deep tenderness over low lumbar segments, with palpable step-off at lumbosacral junction; tenderness in bilateral buttocks; standing Trendelenberg test negative bilaterally; range of motion full in forward flexion plane, but limited in extension plane due to increased low back pain; straight leg raise test negative bilaterally; peripheral pulses trace at posterior tibial sites, 1+ at popliteal sites; Fabre's test reveals no localizing pain to hip or buttock region, but does reproduce low back pain on right side.

Laboratory Findings: Lumbar spine radiographs (anteroposterior/lateral and oblique): grade 2 forward slippage of fifth lumbar vertebra off sacrum; L5 pars defects; no instability on flexion-extension views; no evidence of hip joint space narrowing, fracture, or deformity. Lumbar MRI (see figure): bilateral pars defects at L5, with moderate disc space narrowing and secondary L5-S1 neural foraminal stenosis; no evidence of central spinal stenosis. Noninvasive arterial Doppler study: arterial ankle/brachial indices (resting) 0.86 right, 1.0 left. Lower extremity electrodiagnostic studies: spontaneous activity (PSW 1+) in bilateral lumbar paraspinals; normal nerve conduction.

Question: What is the cause of this patient's leg pain?

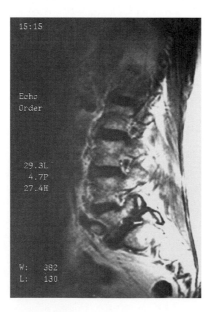

Answer: Neurogenic claudication secondary to L5-S1 grade 2 isthmic spondylolisthesis with secondary neuroforaminal stenosis

Discussion: The term spondylolisthesis was first used by Killan in 1854 and is derived from the Greek words *spondylos* (vertebra) and *olisthy* (to slip or slide). The condition has come to be recognized as a heterogeneous group of spinal disorders that share the common feature of forward displacement of one spinal segment upon another. The radiologic classification system of Meyerding is used widely to quantify the degree of slip with respect to the next inferior vertebral body. Grades I–IV describe the percent forward slippage. Grade I is a 0-25% forward slip, grade II is a 25-50% slip, grade III is a 50-75% slip, grade IV is a 75-100% slip, and grade V is more than 100% slippage (also known as spondyloptosis).

Wiltse and Rothman authored the most comprehensive description of the various types of lesions resulting in spondylolisthesis. Each type describes a variation of failure of the posterior elements, resulting in an inability of the affected segment to resist anterior shear stress, so that forward displacement occurs.

Type I—congenital/dysplastic. This type is characterized by dysplasia of the facet joint of the upper sacrum, which leads to an inability to resist shear stresses, and forward slippage occurs. Subtypes describe the particular congenital abnormality. Subtype A describes axially oriented articular processes; subtype B describes the sagitally orientation; and subtype C describes all other congenital deformities.

Type II—isthmic. Lesions of the pars interarticularis characterize this type. Subtype A describes a fracture of the pars, usually a stress fracture due to congenital weakness. Subtype B describes elongated pars due to repeated cracking and healing of the stress fracture over time.

Type III—degenerative. This type is characterized by intersegmental instability due to long standing disc space degeneration.

Type IV—pathologic. This type is characterized by a traumatically induced lesion or fracture of the posterior elements in an area other than the pars interarticularis (i.e., pedicle or facet).

Type V—pathologic. This type is due to metabolic bone disease that results in an isthmic defect or an elongated but intact pars.

Type VI—postsurgical. This type is due to loss of posterior support structures secondary to surgical decompression.

The most common clinical presentation is of the isthmic type. Involvement occurs most often at L5-S1 at 82.1%, followed by L4-L5 at 11.3%, then L3-L4 at 0.5%, and L2-L3 at 0.3%. There is a preference in sex and race: Caucasian men have the highest incidence (6.4%), and African-American women having the lowest (1.1%). Physical exertion and competitive sports, which induce stressed hyperextension and rotation, seem to be causative factors. The subgroup with the highest prevalence is weightlifters at 36%. Others at risk include college football linemen, gymnasts, judoists, new army recruits, javelin throwers, pole-vaulters, loggers, and adolescents with thoracolumbar osteochondrosis. The condition is seemingly limited to those with upright posture, with a low occurrence in neuromuscular nonambulators. Most cases develop in the first year of school, and by age 7 the incidence is 4%. Another 1.4% of cases develop during adolescence.

Clinical pain presentation in spondylolisthesis is most commonly one of activity-induced mechanical lower back pain. The lesion itself is most likely the cause of the symptoms in the young adult; the spondylolisthesis and the biomechanical factors associated therewith are most likely the causes of pain in the third, fourth and fifth decades. As disc degeneration progresses, it becomes the primary source of low back pain. The location and character of the symptoms combined with selective diagnostic injections and discography can aide in the accurate diagnosis of the primary pain generator. The pars has been shown to have free nerve endings and therefore can be considered a source of pain; however, it is unlikely to be the *only* source of pain—especially in the subacute and chronic stages of this condition.

Radicular pain, as seen in this patient, is relatively uncommon and represents only 14% of case presentations. Causes of radiculopathy include disc herniation at or adjacent to the level of the listhesis, fibrocartilagenous overgrowth of the pars defect, stretching of the nerve root due to forward vertebral slippage, and lateral nerve root entrapment due to foraminal narrowing, as in the present patient.

Progression of the listhesis in adult life is possible, but uncommon, possibly due to spinal soft tissue support (i.e., ligament and disc) and as well as paraspinal muscular contraction. Degeneration of the disc space may also provide segmental stabilization. Instability is greater at the L4-L5 level, which may progress into the third or fourth decades of life. If the listhesis is less than 10%, there is little risk for low back pain. For listhesis over 25%, the incidence of low back pain increases, and there is earlier evidence of degenerative disc disease in comparison to the general population.

Treatment of lumbar spondylolisthesis begins with education and reassurance of the patient regarding the condition. The biomechanical implications of their typical activities must be understood and work tasks modified to avoid repetitive hyperextension and rotation, at least in symptomatic individuals. Therapeutic exercise favors a flexion-biased approach that includes abdominal strengthening, pelvic tilt, and knee-to-chest stretching. Reducing lordotic shear by minimizing and/or stabilizing lumbar lordosis has been shown to aid in control of pain. The use of a lumbosacral orthosis in low-grade slippage has been shown to significantly reduce pain. Additional conservative options include medications to control pain and inflammation, mobilization and manipulation, traction (preferably 90/90 supine positioning), and selective spinal injections. Surgical treatment becomes a reasonable option if pain becomes intolerable or, more certainly, if progressive neurologic deficit develops.

Although the present patient had a history of vascular claudication, her ankle/arm indexes were not severe enough to suggest this as the source of her leg symptoms. Furthermore, the pattern of pain on standing alone did not support arterial occlusion as the cause. Initial conservative treatment offered included biomechanical counseling, a home exercise program emphasizing flexion-biased exercises, and pharmacologic control of pain and inflammation. External stabilization with a modified Boston double-overlap lumbosacral orthosis improved her back pain with activities, but did nothing to control her radicular pain. Periodic transforaminal epidural steroid injections were of temporary benefit initially, but the relief period shortened as time went on. This patient had adequate control of symptoms with conservative care for almost 5 years. Due to progressive pain and functional limitation, she ultimately elected to undergo decompressive laminectomy with L5-S1 interbody fusion and posterior instrumentation. The outcome was successful.

Clinical Pearls

1. Both standing and walking aggravate claudication of neurogenic origin. In contrast, vascular claudication is aggravated by walking alone (i.e., activity-induced oxygen depletion).

2. The patient's pattern of pain (i.e., leg versus back and flexion versus extension intolerance) is more informative in determining the cause of pain than the finding of spondylolysis or spondylolisthesis on a radiograph. Augment your history and physical exam with selective diagnostic injections and/or discography to confirm the primary pain generator.

3. Radiculopathy is an uncommon manifestation of spondylolisthesis. Due to the disconnection between the posterior neural arch and the vertebral body, it is uncommon to see central spinal stenosis associated with spondylolisthesis. Neuroforaminal stenosis at the level of the listhesis is a common and frequently overlooked cause of radiculopathy in these patients.

REFERENCES

1. Grobler LJ, Wiltse LL: The Adult Spine Principles and Practice, 2nd ed. Philadelphia, Lippincott-Raven Publishers, 1997, pp 1865–1921.
2. Meyerding HW: Spondylolisthesis. Surg Gynecol Obstet 54: 371–377, 1932.
3. Steiner ME, Micheli LJ: Treatment of symptomatic spondylolysis and spondylolisthesis with the modified Boston brace. Spine 10:937–943, 1985.
4. Wiltse LL, Rothman LG: Spondylolisthesis: Classification, diagnosis, and natural history. Semin Spine Surg 1(2): 78–94, 1989.

PATIENT 8

A 65-year-old woman with left shoulder pain

A 65-year-old, right-handed woman presents with a 3-day history of left shoulder swelling, pain, and decreased motion. She was moving furniture the night before the onset of these complaints. She denies fever, chills, and other musculoskeletal or neurologic symptoms, and describes the pain as sharp, stabbing, and radiating to the proximal arm. There is no numbness, but she is unable to lift her left arm. There is no significant past history.

Physical Examination: Musculoskeletal: swelling and tenderness of left shoulder anteriorly, no erythema or warmth; inability to initiate a flexion-abduction arc; strength assessment difficult secondary to pain. Cervical spine: normal. Neurologic: normal.

Laboratory Findings: Hemorrhagic shoulder aspiration, with normal white cell count. X-rays: mild degenerative glenohumeral and acromioclvicular disease; no evidence of fracture or dislocation. MRI: see figures.

Question: What is the diagnosis?

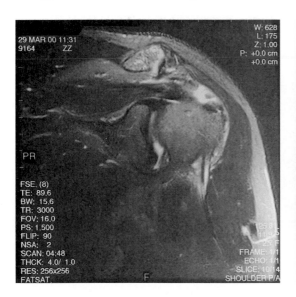 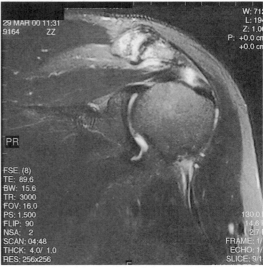

Diagnosis: Complete rotator cuff tear.

Discussion: Rotator cuff failure is a common shoulder disorder in clinical practice. It can be categorized as partial or full thickness, acute or chronic, and traumatic or degenerative. The most common site of tear is near the attachment of the cuff to the tuberosities, and the tear nearly always begins in the supraspinatus part of the cuff near the bicipital tendon. Most full-thickness tears occur in a tendon that is weakened by repeated small episodes of trauma, steroid injections, subacromial impingement, hypovascularity of the tendon, major trauma, and/or previous partial tears. Complete rotator cuff tears are uncommon prior to age 40, even with the most massive injuries. Dislocations or bony failure is common in these younger individuals.

Neer has suggested that physical examination may not be reliable in differentiating chronic bursitis and partial tears from complete tears. Look for bursal effusions, palpable cuff defect, muscle atrophy, pain on shoulder elevation, and more passive than active range of motion on clinical evaluations. **Decreased external rotation strength** is one of the most sensitive indicators of the magnitude of the tear.

Plain x-rays, obtained to rule out any bony problems, generally are normal. Ultrasonography provides a noninvasive means of diagnosis, but it is operator dependent. Shoulder arthrography is the standard investigative technique for diagnosis, but it is invasive, and contrast material in the glenohumeral joint leaks into the subacromial bursa. Nevertheless, MRI and CT arthrograms are the usual images examined.

Arthroscopic examination is also recommended to check for other, associated bony abnormalities. Differential diagnoses to consider are traumatic bursitis, shoulder dislocation, inflammatory diseases, acromioclavicular separation, and C5-6 disc disease.

When treating a rotator cuff failure, it is essential to know that tears are not always painful and do not always cause dysfunction. Aggressive treatment is indicated only in symptomatic patients. Goals of treatment are restoration of comfort, restoration of function, and prevention of future problems. Nonoperative treatment should be recommended for at least 4–6 weeks, before making a decision for surgery. **Conservative regimens** have claimed success in about 30–40% of patients. Surgical repair results are good to excellent in approximately 80%. Note that extensive postoperative rehabilitation is required. Major causes of surgical failure are infection, deltoid denervation, deltoid detachment, adhesions, failure of the repair, and inadequate subacromial decompression.

In the present patient, MRI revealed complete rotator cuff tear with degenerative changes. Conservative management over 10 weeks was unsuccessful; she had persistent pain, restriction of movements, and decreased strength. A repair of the rotator cuff was performed. Subsequently, the patient was free of pain and regained at least 80% of her usual shoulder movements. Her strength showed continued improvement at early follow-up.

Clinical Pearls

1. Complete rotator cuff tears are uncommon prior to age 40, even in the most massive injuries.

2. Decreased external rotation strength is one of the most sensitive indicators of the magnitude of the tear.

3. Differential diagnoses to consider are traumatic bursitis, shoulder dislocation, inflammatory diseases, acromioclavicular separation, and C5–6 disc disease.

4. Recommend nonoperative treatment for at least 4–6 weeks, before a decision is made for surgery. Conservative regimens have claimed success in about 30–40% of patients.

REFERENCES

1. Gartsman GM, Taverna E: The incidence of glenohumeral joint abnormalities associated with full-thickness, reparable rotator cuff tears. Arthroscopy 13: 450–455, 1997.
2. Naviaser RJ: Tears of the rotator cuff. Orthoped Clin North Am 11: 295–306, 1980.
3. Neer CS, Craig EV, Fakuda H: Rotator cuff arthropathy. J Bone Joint Surg Am 65:1232–1244, 1983.
4. Rokito AS, Cuomo F, Gallagher MA, Zuckerman JD: Long-term functional outcome of repair of large and massive chronic tears of the rotator cuff. J Bone Joint Surg Am 81:991–997, 1999.

PATIENT 9

A 35-year-old woman with left hand pain and swelling

A 35-year-old woman presents with a history of a minimally displaced fracture of her left radial shaft 12 weeks ago. The fracture was treated successfully with closed reduction and immobilization. One week after removal of her cast, the patient began experiencing burning pain, swelling, and patchy numbness involving the left wrist, hands, and fingers. She was initially treated with nonsterioidal anti-inflammatory drugs (NSAIDs). Little improvement was seen after 1 week. As symptoms persisted, NSAIDs were discontinued, and the patient was placed on a tapering course of oral prednisone. Two weeks after steroids had begun, the patient began to complain of intermittent nausea, abdominal pain, and dark-colored stools.

Physical Examination: Vital signs: normal. Temperature of hands: left 29.5° C, right 32° C. Musculoskeletal: active range of motion (ROM) decreased in left hand, with 2nd through 5th metacarpophalangeal flexion 70%, 2nd through 5th proximal interphalangeal flexion 80%; wrist ulnar and radial deviation 25% and 15%, respectively; passive ROM preserved in hand, fingers, and wrist; passive ROM elbow flexion and extension and shoulder flexion, extension, and abduction all normal. Skin: mild hyperhidrosis and non-pitting edema on left hand when compared to right. Neurologic: upper extremity reflexes normal in biceps, triceps, and brachioradialis bilaterally; accounting for decreases secondary to pain, 4+/5 strength in distal left upper extremity, 5/5 proximally and bilaterally; hyperesthesia (allodynia) and hyperpathia to soft touch; weakness apparently secondary to painful motion; pinprick and two-point discrimination normal.

Laboratory Findings: CBC: mildly increased WBCs (14,000/µl); normal differential; hemoglobin 12, Hct 39. Electrolytes and ESR: normal. ANA: negative. Urinalysis: normal. Hemoccult: positive. Nerve conduction studies: left median motor—onset latency 3.5 msec, conduction velocity 58 mps; left median sensory—orthodromically to middle finger peak latency of 3.0 msec, amplitude 17 mcv; left ulnar motor—latency 3 msec at wrist and 7.9 msec at elbow, conduction velocity 59 m/sec and 53 m/sec at elbow. Plain radiographs of left hand: no fractures or osteopenia.

Question: What is the diagnosis?

Answers: Complex regional pain syndrome (CRPS) type I and steroid-induced gastritis

Discussion: Treatment of CRPS is both controversial and challenging. Physical and psychological impairment often coexist. Better outcomes have been achieved with early diagnosis and treatment. Treatments include physical therapy with general modalities, massage, and active and passive range of motion in which the goal is to improve functional movement. Some studies report corticosteroids to be highly effective, although the efficacy of NSAIDs has not been as favorable. Electrical stimulation involving the spinal cord or use of transcutaneous electrical nerve stimulation has also met with some success. Other oral medications include anticonvulsants, tricyclic antidepressants, beta blockers, and tranquilizers. Unfortunately, most treatments are based on clinical assumptions and impressions, as controlled research on these therapies is lacking. Sympathetic blocks are often used when other therapies fail. Multiple blocks are often needed, and long-term relief is a rarity. Opponents of sympathetic blocks assert that when studies were stringently controlled for placebo, no relief attributable to the block was found. Lastly, patients often require psychological counseling and behavior management due to anxiety and depression.

The physiologic action of steroids in treating CRPS is unknown. Steroids, however, are often used in the acute stage to treat symptoms that appear to be an inflammatory process. The anti-inflammatory properties of steroids are mediated at the cellular and vascular level. Capillary dilatation and permeability are reduced, and leukocyte function is decreased. Therefore, inflammatory processes mediated by vasoactive kinins are reduced.

Corticosteroids unfortunately have been linked to an increased incidence of peptic ulcer. GI side effects usually only develop when treatment duration is longer than 30 day, or when the total dose of prednisone exceeds 1 g. Other possible GI side effects from steroids are pancreatitis, abdominal distention, and ulcerative esophagitis. Transient increases in liver enzymes are often noted with steroid use.

Systemic side effects of corticosteroid use are well documented. Some of the more common include carbohydrate intolerance with manifestation of latent diabetes mellitus, hyperlipidemia, and fluid and electrolyte disorders. Symptoms of congestive heart failure may also worsen. Some CNS side effects include insomnia, restlessness, agitation, and depression. Dermatologically, impaired wound healing or facial flushing may occur. Prolonged therapy (for more than 2 months) often results in features of Cushing's syndrome. Chronic high doses always result in pituitary-adrenal suppression and serious immune consequences.

Fortunately, there are other therapies for CRPS to explore when steroids aren't tolerated.

Clinical Pearls

1. Favorable outcomes in complex regional pain syndrome (CRPS) type I depend on early diagnosis and treatment to prevent symptoms from becoming chronic.
2. Oral corticosteroid therapy is often used in the early treatment of CRPS.
3. GI side effects are common with prolonged use of corticosteroids.
4. Treatment of CRPS also includes physical therapy to increase functional range of motion, electrical stimulation, multiple sympathetic blocks, and, in some cases, surgical sympathectomy.

REFERENCES

1. Kasdan ML, Johnson AL: Reflex sympathetic dystrophy. Occup Med 13(3) 521–531, 1998.
2. Lennard TA, Shin D: Physiatric Procedures in Clinical Practice. Philadelphia, Hanley & Belfus, Inc., 1995.

PATIENT 10

A 35-year-old woman with pain and swelling of both knees

A 35-year-old woman noticed right knee pain of insidious onset about 3 months ago. The knee usually becomes painful and swollen after prolonged weight-bearing, and the pain diminishes after she takes over-the-counter anti-inflammatory medicine and rests the knee. Now, she notices similar pain and swelling in the other knee. She denies chills, rash, or GI symptoms, but has had a low-grade fever for the past couple of days. Her only other complaint is pain and swelling in her right elbow after a long day of gardening. Past medical history is significant for seasonal allergies, for which she takes an antihistamine.

Physical Examination: Temperature 99.5°, pulse 90, respirations 16, blood pressure 125/75 mmHg. General: normal weight for height and age. HEENT: mild erythema with clear mucus in oral cavity; increased erythema of the sclera, pupils equal and react to light and accomodation; lymph nodes normal, nontender. Skin: no rash or lesion. Chest: clear, without wheezes. Cardiac: normal. Abdomen: normal. Extremities: tender and swollen over medial and lateral joint lines of both knees; range of motion normal, but with increased pain at > 120 degrees flexion; negative McMurry; normal drawer; no crepitus. Right elbow tender and swollen mainly at medial epicondyle; range of motion normal.

Laboratory Findings: WBC 10,500/µl; Hct 41%; platelets 375,000/µl. Differential: normal, except eosinophils slightly elevated. Erythrocyte sedimentation rate: 45 (normal 0-30 mm/hr). Urinalysis: normal. X-rays of knees (*see figure; anteroposterior view of right knee shown*): medial and lateral joint space narrowing in both knees; periarticular osteoporosis; no evidence of bony repair. X-ray of right elbow: periarticular osteoporosis.

Question: What laboratory study would be most helpful in making the diagnosis?

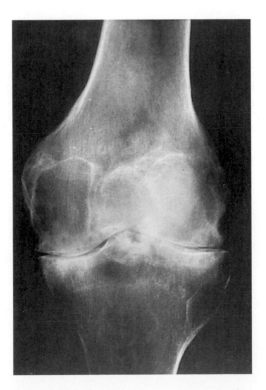

Answer: Rheumatoid factor

Discussion: Rheumatoid arthritis (RA) does not always present with signs and symptoms in the distal extremities. In some patients, the presenting symptoms may be in the more proximal joints such as the knees, elbows, or shoulders. RA is defined as a systemic inflammatory disorder involving multiple joints and support structures. It is a **symmetric polyarthritis** that affects synovial joints, primarily the hands, wrists, elbows, shoulders, feet, ankles, and knees. The exact cause of the inflammatory process is unknown, but it involves dysregulated production of cytokines. Studies suggest that both genetic and environmental factors may be involved. RA is most prevalent between the fourth and fifth decades, and affects women two to three times more often than men.

The pathophysiology involves the proliferation of cells (macrophages and fibroblasts) that line the synovial tissues. Microvascular injury results from microthrombi and inflammatory cell infiltration. As the disease progresses, the inflamed synovial tissue produces several cytokines and enzymes that invade the joints and cause degradation of hyaline cartilage and bone; this results in **joint space loss** and **marginal joint erosions**.

The American College of Rheumatology diagnostic criteria for RA include morning joint stiffness, symmetrical presentation, polyarticular inflammation, rheumatoid nodules, serum rheumatoid factor, and radiographic evidence of marginal joint erosions and/or **periarticular osteoporosis**.

Treatment for RA involves pharmacologic therapy, physical therapy, prevention, rest, and judicious use of surgery. The four classes of medications used to treat RA are: NSAIDS, analgesics, glucocorticoids, and disease-modifying antirheumatic drugs (DMARDs). Recently, the number of drugs in the latter class has expanded (for a detailed discussion and comprehensive review of DMARDs, see Schuna and Megeff). Traditional pharmacologic treatment for RA involved a "treatment pyramid," which started with education at the top, then the initiation of NSAIDs, often followed by glucocorticoids prior to, or in conjunction with, DMARDs. However, the contemporary trend is to use the "reverse pyramid," in which DMARDs are initiated during the early stages of the disease and often in combination; they are followed by glucocorticoids and NSAIDs.

The traditional philosophy about exercise in patients with RA emphasized avoiding isotonic exercises in the presence of inflamed joints; the focus was on isometric exercise for these patients. The goal was to rest inflamed joints to avoid acceleration of joint destruction. Recent studies have shown that **dynamic weight-bearing exercises** can improve joint mobility, muscle strength, and aerobic conditioning. There is *no* evidence that vigorous exercise exacerbates the arthritis or causes progression in radiologically documented damage. In addition, dynamic resistance strength training in patients with RA can reduce pain and fatigue and improve functional status.

The present patient's rheumatoid factor was 174, and the x-ray of her right elbow revealed periarticular osteoporosis and joint space narrowing. Her family doctor referred her to a rheumatologist, who confirmed the diagnosis of RA and started her on a combination treatment of low-dose oral prednisone and leflunomide (Arava); the latter inhibits the synthesis of pyrimidines and interferes with the production of immune cells. (The rheumatologist attributed the low-grade fever, elevated white blood cell count, and positive HEENT findings to a sinus infection.) The patient was enrolled in an aqua therapy program, which provided the strengthening and conditioning benefits of the exercise as well as the therapeutic effects of the warm water. After her flare-up stabilized, she tapered off the prednisone and replaced it with celecoxib, a COX-2 selective inhibitor, in addition to the Arava. She has been able to minimize occasional additions of prednisone to her drug regimen, and is maintaining a productive lifestyle.

Clinical Pearls

1. Rheumatoid arthritis does not always present with signs and symptoms in joints of the distal extremities; initial findings may be in the knees, shoulders, or elbows.

2. The current trend in pharmacologic management of RA is to institute the disease-modifying antirheumatic drugs earlier in the disease course, often in combination.

3. Recent studies have shown that dynamic weight-bearing exercise can improve joint mobility, muscle strength, and aerobic conditioning.

4. There is no evidence that vigorous exercise exacerbates RA, or causes progression in the radiologically documented damage.

REFERENCES

1. Goldring SR: A 55-year-old woman with rheumatoid arthritis. JAMA. 283(4):524–531, 2000.
2. Hazes JMW, van den Ende CHM:. How vigorously should we exercise our rheumatoid arthritis patients? Ann Rheum Dis 55(12):861–862, 1996.
3. Mikuls JR, O'Dell J: The changing face of RA therapy: Results of serial surveys. Arth Rheum 43(2):464–465, 2000.
4. Noreau L, Moffet H, et al: Dance-based exercise program in rheumatoid arthritis: Feasability in individuals with American College of Rheumatology Functional Class III Disease. Am J Phys Med Rehabil 76(2):109–113, 1997.
5. Schuna AA, Megeff C: New drugs for the treatment of RA. Am J Health-System Pharm 57(3):225–234, 2000.

PATIENT 11

A 42-year-old woman with left shoulder and neck pain

A 42-year-old, right-handed woman presents with a 10-year history of nagging, persistent left shoulder and neck pain. Her problem began insidiously without other symptoms—only a nagging, dull ache and a sensation of muscle tightness and "spasm" in the area between the shoulder and neck. She relates the severity of pain at about 4–5 (10 = worst pain) on most days. Certain activities aggravate her problem: driving, left-handed movements, typing, and gardening. Pain is relieved with sleep, but worse under periods of stress. She denies radiation of pain, sensory disturbances, or other central nervous system problems. Previous treatment involving trigger point injections into the neck and back was unsuccessful. Similarly, muscle relaxants were not helpful in relieving painful spasms. Past medical history appears to be noncontributory. Family history is unknown.

Physical Examination: General: well-nourished, well-developed; no distress. HEENT: pupils equally round and reactive; neck supple, without masses. Neurologic: reflexes, gait, and cranial nerves normal. Musculoskeletal: Spurling's test normal; decreased range-of-motion in cervical rotation to left compared to right; markedly enlarged left upper trapezius muscle visible when compared to contralateral shoulder (see figure); thickened, tight left upper trapezius muscle, without trigger points.

Laboratory Findings: Nerve conduction and EMG study of both upper limbs: continuous motor unit firing (abnormal muscle contraction) of left upper trapezius muscle, even when patient attempts to relax; similar findings in left sternoclaidomastoid muscle.

Question: What procedure might be most effective in reducing pain in this condition?

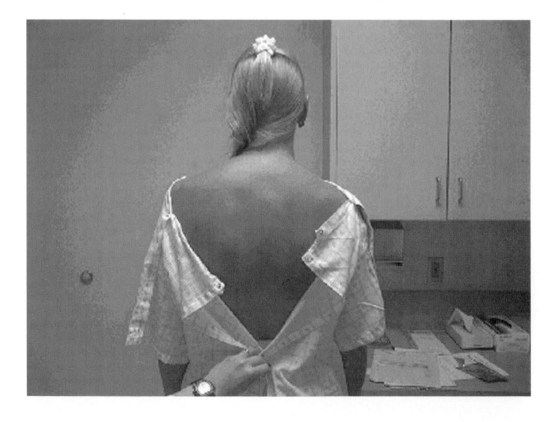

Answer: Botulinum toxin injection

Discussion: This case illustrates an unusual presentation of focal dystonia, fic confirmatory laboratory test to make such a diagnosis, EMG findings may be helpful to identify the specific muscle or muscles that are involved.

Botulinum toxin type A (BTX-A) has been reported to be effective in treating focal dystonias. (BTX-A is licensed for use in the U.S. for the treatment of blepharospasm, strabismus, and hemifacial spasm.) In this case, local injection of 50 units of BTX-A into the left upper trapezius resulted in dramatic reduction in pain and spasm within 1 week. EMG guidance was used to carefully identify the abnormally contracting muscle, and the injections were made at specific points (see figure, *arrows*). A dual-purpose EMG recording needle with a port adapted for simultaneous injection was employed.

Clinical Pearls

1. The onset of focal dystonia is generally insidious. Symptoms may be worsened under periods of stress or when performing certain physical activities. A history of abrupt onset, bilateral symptoms, and lack of relief with onset of sleep is not generally considered consistent with a diagnosis of focal dystonia.

2. Pain is often associated with focal dystonia. Botulinum toxin treatment shows promise as an effective treatment for some painful conditions involving skeletal muscle.

3. The initial diagnosis and treatment of dystonia should be made in conjunction with a movement disorders specialist (neurologist) trained in the management of such conditions.

REFERENCES
1. Childers MK: Use of Botulinum Toxin Type A in Pain Management. New York, DEMOS Medical Publishing, 1999.
2. Fahn S: The varied clinical expressions of dystonia. Neurol Clin 2(3): 541–544, 1984.
3. Grandas F: Clinical application of botulinum toxin. [Spanish] Neurologia 10:224–233, 1995.
4. Kelleher JF, Mandell AJ: Dystonia musculorum deformans: A "critical phenomenon" model involving nigral dopaminergic and caudate pathways. [review] Medical Hypotheses 31(1):55–88, 1990.
5. Markham CH: The dystonias. [review] Curr Opini Neurol Neurosurg 5(3):301–377, 1992.

PATIENT 12

A 79-year-old man with poor balance

A 79-year-old man presents with complaints of poor balance, which started 9 months prior to the evaluation. Almost immediately after his problems with balance began, he noticed numbness and tingling in his feet and fingers that gradually progressed to include his wrists and knees. Subsequently, weakness in his legs developed, causing him to need a walker for ambulation. His weakness continued to worsen, and for the last 3 months he has required a wheelchair for community ambulation, but continued to use the walker for household ambulation. He has also noticed weakness in his hands and loss of muscle bulk. He denies any bowel or bladder symptoms.

Physical Examination: Extremities: weakness in all extremities, with legs more affected than arms; in each limb, distal muscles more affected than proximal ones. Neurologic: deep tendon reflexes absent; loss of pin-prick, vibration, and proprioception in stocking-glove configuration.

Laboratory Findings: See results of nerve conduction and EMG studies below.

Question: Do the study results point to a specific diagnosis?

Nerve Conduction Study

Nerve	Site	Latency	CV	Amplitude	F wave
R Median (m)	Wrist-APB	14.1 ms		2.59 mV	135.7 ms
	Elbow-wrist		12.8 m/s	1.88 mV	
R Ulnar (m)	Wrist-ADM	11.6 ms		3.02 mV	NR
	Below elb-wrist		12.3 m/s	0.28 mV	
	Above elb-below elb	10.0 m/s		0.20 mV	
R Tibial (m)	Ankle-AH	NR			
R Peroneal (m)	FH-Tib Ant	NR			
R Ulnar (s)	Wrist-dig V	NR			
R Radial (s)	Wrist-dig I	NR			
R Median (s)	Wrist-dig III	NR			
Sural (s)	Mid-calf-ankle	NR			

(m) = motor, (s) = sensory, CV = conduction velocity, APB = abductor pollicis brevis, ADM = abductor digiti minimi, AH = abductor hallucis, FH = fibular head, NR = no response, m/s = meters/second

EMG Study

Muscle	Fibs	PSWs	Fascic	MUAP dur	MUAP amp	MUAP config	Int Pat
R Tib Ant	3+	3+	0	nl	nl	nl	Very red
R Med Gastr	3+	3+	0	nl	nl	nl	Very red
R Vast Lat	1+	1+	0	inc	nl	polyphasic	Mod red
R FDI	2+	2+	0	inc	large	polyphasic	Mild red
R EDC	1+	1+	0	inc	nl	polyphasic	Mild red

Fibs = fibrillations, PSW = positive sharp waves, MUAP = motor unit action potential, Int Pat = interference pattern, Tib Ant = tibialis anterior, Med Gastr = medial gastrocnemius, Vast Lat = vastus lateralis, FDI = first dorsal interosseous, EDC = extensor digitorum communis, nl = normal, inc = increased, red = reduced

Diagnosis: Chronic inflammatory demyelinating polyneuropathy

Discussion: Based on the evidence from the clinical examination, electrodiagnostic evidence of a polyneuropathy would be expected. Unlike the clinical exam, nerve conduction studies (NCS) can assist with the differentiation between a polyneuropathy due primarily to a demyelinating process and an axonal one. This distinction is particularly important because the etiologies of and therapy for the two processes differ significantly. In this case, there is marked prolongation of motor distal latencies and slowing of nerve conduction velocities in the upper extremities. The median F-wave latency is dramatically prolonged. A proximal conduction block, most prominent in the segment of the ulnar nerve between the wrist and elbow, is present. A conduction block on NCS is defined by a loss of amplitude of greater than 20% when comparing proximal to distal stimulation results. A notable exception for the tibial nerve must be recognized, because a 50% drop in amplitude may occur as a normal finding with electrical stimulation of the nerve in the popliteal fossa compared to stimulation at the ankle.

The process in the present patient is primarily a demyelinating one, with a secondary axonal loss. **Hallmark features of a demyelination process are:**

- Conduction block
- Temporal dispersion
- Prolongation of distal latencies
- Slowing of conduction velocities
- Prolongation or absence of F waves.

If the lesion is purely demyelinating, spontaneous activity is absent on electromyography (EMG), and motor units action potentials are normal in appearance. A loss of amplitude on NCS may be due to either a secondary axonal loss or distal conduction block. The presence of denervation changes on EMG needle examination suggests axonal loss. A normal EMG exam (except for possible reduction in the interference pattern) suggests a distal conduction block.

This patient also has **evidence of secondary axonal loss:**

- Absence of sensory nerve action potentials
- Absence of right tibial and peroneal compound muscle action potentials (CMAP)
- Reduction of the amplitude of the right median and ulnar CMAP
- Changes on EMG consistent with acute denervation and chronic reinnervation changes
- Involvement of both sensory and motor fibers demonstrated on NCS.

Much has been published on the electrophysiologic criteria for demyelinating neuropathy and for differentiating between acute and chronic processes. The acquired demyelinating neuropathies are commonly immune-mediated and have other clinical correlates of those disorders. Occasionally, patients may have a gammopathy or an antibody to myelin-associated glycoprotein. Demyelinating neuropathies may also be seen in diabetes mellitus, with certain toxins (including arsenic), and in HIV.

In the present patient, the clinical features together with the NCS/EMG support the diagnosis of chronic inflammatory demyelinating polyneuropathy. The patient, with exception of an elevated CSF protein of 150, had normal laboratory values.

Clinical Pearls

1. In inherited demyelinating neuropathies, conduction block and temporal dispersion are typically absent, and conduction velocities show little variation between nerves or segments.

2. Submaximal proximal stimulation and Martin-Grubler anastomosis may mimic conduction block.

3. In acute demyelinating neuropathy, if the patient is studied soon after symptom onset, prolongation of F wave latencies may be the earliest and only finding.

REFERENCES

1. Albers JW, Kelly JJ: Acquired inflammatory demyelinating polyneuropathies: Clinical and electrodiagnositic features. Muscle Nerve 12:435–451, 1989.
2. Bouchard C, Lacroix C, et al: Clinicopathologic findings and prognosis in chronic inflammatory demyelinating polyneuropathy. Neurology 52:498–503, 1999.
3. Bromberg MB: Comparison of electrodiagnositic criteria for primary demyelination in chronic polyneuropathy. Muscle Nerve 14(10):968–976, 1991.
4. Donofrio P, Albers J: AAEM minimonograph #34: Polyneuropathy: Classification by nerve conduction studies and electromyography. Muscle Nerve 13:889–903, 1990.
5. Lewis RA, Sumner AJ: The electrodiagnostic distinctions between chronic familial and acquired demyelinating neuropathies. Neurology 32:592–596, 1982.

PATIENT 13

A 24-year-old man with acute subdural hematoma and hallucinations

A 24-year-old man after suffered a blow on the head during an altercation, and a subdural hematoma developed in his left temporal area. His initial Glasgow Coma Scale score was 3 (eyes–1, motor–1, verbal–1). He was in a coma for 16 days. Over the next 4 weeks, he showed gradual improvement in alertness and awareness. He then started saying that he smelled burning leaves inside his hospital room intermittently during the day.

Physical Exam: Blood pressure 110/60, pulse 90, respiration 16, temperature 97.9°. General: no acute cardiorespiratory distress. HEENT, heart, lungs, and abdomen: normal. Neurologic: alert; oriented to self only; poor short-term and long-term memory; no agitation; muscle strength 5/5; sensation and reflexes intact. Gait: mildly ataxic

Laboratory Findings: WBC 9300 /µl, Hct 45%, platelets 266,000/µl. Electrolytes: Na^+ 140 mEq/L, K^+ 5 mEq/L, Cl^- 100 mEq/L, HCO_3^- 26 mEq/L. BUN 11 mg/dl, creatinine 1 mg/dl. EEG: see figure.

Question: What is the cause of the patient's hallucinations?

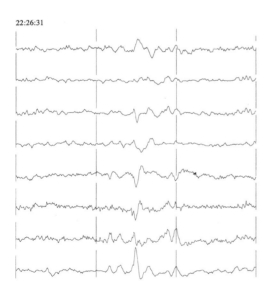

Left Hemisphere EEG

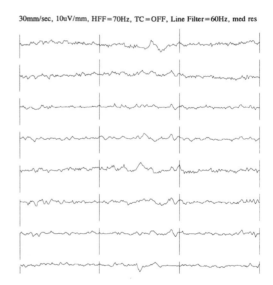

Right Hemisphere EEG

Answer: Post-traumatic simple partial seizures

Discussion: The risk of post-traumatic seizures increases with the severity of injury. A post-traumatic seizure is defined as an initial or recurrent seizure episode, not attributable to another obvious cause, after penetrating or non-penetrating traumatic brain injury (TBI), and it refers to both single and recurrent episodes. A post-traumatic seizure is classified as immediate (within 24 hours of TBI), early (within 1 week of TBI), or late (more than 1 week after TBI). Post-traumatic epilepsy is a term reserved for *recurrent*, late post-traumatic seizure.

The diagnosis of post-traumatic seizure can be difficult. Actual observation of the seizure activity may provide the best information. An electroencephalogram (EEG) can help support the diagnosis by showing spike and sharp waves, as in the present patient's tracing. An elevated serum prolactin level also supports the diagnosis of post-traumatic seizure, but a normal level does not rule it out.

Simple partial seizures are frequently referred to as auras, and may manifest as abnormal sensation (e.g., flashing lights, smells), or experimental phenomenon (e.g., déjà vu). Partial seizures can be treated with a variety of anticonvulsants, such as carbamazepine, gabapentin, lamotrigine, phenobarbital, phenytoin, and primidone.

Clinical Pearls

1. The relative risk of recurrent seizures is highest among patients with a history of prolonged coma (i.e., more than 7 days), and acute subdural hematoma.

2. A late post-traumatic seizure is defined as a seizure that occurs more than 1 week after a traumatic brain injury.

3. Post-traumatic epilepsy refers to late, *recurrent* seizures.

4. An elevated serum prolactin level can help support the diagnosis of post-traumatic seizure, but a normal level does not exclude the possibility of seizures.

REFERENCES

1. Brain Injury Special Interest Group of the American Academy of Physical Medicine and Rehabilitation: Practice Parameter: Antiepileptic drug treatment of post-traumatic seizures. Arch Phys Med Rehabil 79:594–597, 1998.
2. Haltiner AM, Temkin NR, Dikmen SS: Risk of seizure recurrence after the first late post-traumatic seizure. Arch Phys Med Rehabil 78:835–840, 1997.
3. Rolak LA (ed): Neurology Secrets. Philadelphia, Hanley and Belfus, Inc., 1993.
4. Rosenthal M, Griffith ER, Kreutzer JS, Pentland B (eds): Rehabilitation of the Adult and Child with Traumatic Brain Injury, 3rd ed. Philadelphia, FA Davis Co, 1999.

PATIENT 14

A 14-year-old boy with functional motor deterioration

A 14-year-old boy presents for clinic follow-up. His mother complains that he cannot get his right leg up on the bed, is falling more often, and cannot stand still in one place. He drools occasionally and sometimes feels dizzy after taking a few steps. His teachers report that he sleeps in school, and his writing has worsened. The patient suffered head trauma due to abuse at 5 weeks of age and has had right hemiparesis and cognitive deficits. Recently he has become more tangential in thinking and has exhibited odd behaviors. He has been seen by a psychiatrist and is currently on Mellaril 100 mg BID as well as Depakote for his well-controlled seizure disorder. He has a positive family history of schizophreniform disorder. You review the history from past clinic visits and note that the problem with falling has gradually worsened over about a year, with an increase in drooling over about 6 months. Mellaril was first started at a dose of 25 mg BID at age 13 and has gradually increased since then.

Physical Examination: General (see figure): height 176.3 cm, weight 78.5 kg, head circumference 58 cm; flat affect with little facial expression. Blood pressure 128/72. Spine: mild lumbar scoliosis that decreases in sitting. Extremities: 1-cm leg length difference (right side shorter); right Trendelenburg in gait; equinovalgus deformity that is not entirely correctable; cogwheeling tremor much more pronounced in right upper extremity; mixed spastic/rigid tone pattern of right lower extremity, somewhat increased in severity since your previous exams; both Babinski's reflexes upgoing.

Laboratory Findings: CT head scan: no change in previously noted areas of encephalomalacia (frontal, temporal, and parietal, and left occipital); prominent ventricles probably due to atrophy. Spine x-rays: 10° levoscoliosis and minimal left hip subluxation. Valproic acid 80; SGOT, SGPT, and CBC normal.

Course: His psychiatrist agrees to reduce the dosage of Mellaril, and the patient is indeed less sleepy on 50 mg q AM and 75 mg q PM. You refer him for serial casting and an orthopedic evaluation; surgery is not recommended. However, he misses the next follow-up in your clinic. When you see him several months later, he has been admitted with pyelonephritis, after his mother, who claims to be a nurse, catheterized him with non-sterile technique due to urinary retention. The patient has lost 40 pounds, has been placed on homebound school, and is using a reclining wheelchair his mother bought at a garage sale. He leans over progressively to the right side, needing support to sit and maximal assistance to bear weight. Inpatient evaluation indicates the weight loss is most likely due to progressive difficulty with swallowing. Another head CT scan is again unchanged.

Questions: How do you explain this patient's deterioration? How would you stop this patient's inexorable decline?

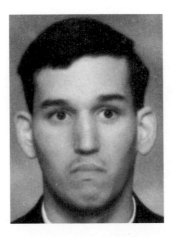

Diagnosis: Drug-induced parkinsonism.

Discussion: This is a classic history for drug-induced parkinsonism. Reducing the dosage of antipsychotic, a medication that this patient needed badly, was not adequate to reverse the syndrome or prevent progression with a cumulative dose over time. The symptom complex of cogwheeling tremor, loss of postural control—especially during activities requiring transitional movement with large shifts of the center of gravity, masked facies, drooling, and dysphagia should never go unrecognized or underestimated.

The syndrome of **tardive dyskinesia**, with severe and disabling oral-facial dystonic posturing, is well known and recognized in previously neurologically intact people after very long-term antipsychotic use. There is also a reaction known as **acute oculogyric crisis** or **dystonic reaction**, which is sudden, severe, and dramatic, and usually occurs shortly after starting medication. **Akathisia** or **restless legs syndrome** is also reported with intermediate-term use.

The parkinsonism syndrome described here seems to be the most commonly observed one in rehabilitation patients, particularly those with brain injury or pathology of any kind, and seems to reverse itself the more quickly it is recognized and the offending medication stopped and/or counteracted. It can be very insidious and sometimes is mistaken for depression or for functional loss related to tightening of contractures with growth. In retrospect, the present patient's symptoms of falling and tightening of contractures, for at least a year, may have been related to Mellaril all along. This author sees several similar cases per year; the usual presenting complaint is marked and unexplained functional deterioration in the presence of known static encephalopathy.

This syndrome is seen even with the newer antipsychotics, such as Risperidone, as well as with Haldol, and may occur or persist in surprisingly low doses in people with pre-existing brain pathology. Prolonged use of drugs may bring about side effects not seen or not as readily apparent or severe on a short course. Several scenarios notoriously can lead to a vicious cycle of giving more and more medication and actually making side effects worse: abdominal pain and Ranitidine; irritability and SSRIs; paradoxical excitement and various sedatives; and, as in this case, worsening "behavior" or decreasing "cooperation" that led to increasing rather than decreasing the dosage over time. Other side effects to beware of in the rehabilitation setting include mental fogginess and anticholinergic side effects on Ditropan; dysphagia, seizures, or hallucinations on baclofen; rashes that can lead to Stevens-Johnson syndrome on anti-epileptic drug levels, particularly phenobarbital, phenytoin, and carbamazepine (usually valproate is the drug of choice if this occurs—cross-reactivity is very high); and dystonia on Reglan, which is similar to tardive dyskinesia.

The best chance of reversing serious side effects quickly and easily is with prompt recognition and reduction or discontinuation. Brief use of sedation or treatment for stress psychosis with Haldol in the intensive care unit is common and may cause only mild to moderate tremor that often resolves without treatment. However, more prolonged stays are not infrequently complicated by full-blown parkinsonism, which requires levodopa and can complicate the proximal weakness due to prolonged neuromusclar blockade common with use of vecuronium or related drugs.

The present patient was given Cogentin and then started on Sinemet 25/100 I tab TID. He received tube feeds for nutritional rehabilitation as part of a successful comprehensive inpatient program to reverse severe deconditioning and return the patient to his previous functional status. Within about 30 days, he was ambulating with orthotic management and eating adequately by mouth. His mother was strongly urged to call the doctor immediately should his function deteriorate again, and to maintain regular clinic visits.

Clinical Pearls

1. Always consider drug side effects, especially when something unusual happens either immediately or some time after starting a new drug. Be aware of well-known side effects. and be prepared to manage them decisively.

2. Never accept functional deterioration without a good explanation.

REFERENCES

1. Akbostanci MC, Atbasoglu EC, Balaban H: Tardive dyskinesia, mild drug-induced dyskinesia, and drug-induced parkinsonism: Risk factors and topographic distribution. Acta Neurol Belg 99(3):176–181, 1999.
2. Caligiuri MP, Lacro JP, Jeste DV: Incidence and predictors of drug-induced parkinsonism in older psychiatric patients treated with very low doses of neuroleptics. J Clin Psychopharmacol 19(4):322–328, 1999.
3. Luchins DJ, Jackman H, Meltzer HY: Lateral ventricular size and drug-induced Parkinsonism. Psychiatry Res 9(1):9–16, 1983.
4. Saltz BL, Woerner MG, Robinson DG, Kane JM: Side effects of antipsychotic drugs: Avoiding and minimizing their impact in elderly patients. Postgrad Med 107(2):169–72, 175–178, 2000.

PATIENT 15

A 27-year-old woman with neck pain after a motor vehicle accident

A 27-year-old woman presents with a 6-month history of neck pain and headache following a motor vehicle accident. The patient was wearing a seatbelt and was driving. It was a rear-end collision with an impact speed estimated at 35 miles per hour. She denies any numbness or tingling in the upper extremities. There is no previous history of any neck pain or headaches prior to this accident. She denies fevers, night sweats, and bowel or bladder incontinence. She reports that some improvement (20–30%) of her symptoms was achieved with physical therapy and oral anti-inflammatories.

Physical Examination: Vital signs: normal. Neurologic: 5/5 strength throughout upper and lower extremities; sensory intact to light touch, pinprick, and propioception; reflexes symmetric bilaterally; long tract signs negative; tenderness in cervical paraspinal musculature at C5-6 level; Spurling and Llhermites signs negative. Musculoskeletal: pain reproduced with extension and rotation of cervical spine.

Laboratory Findings: X-rays: cervical extension, flexion, and rotation restricted due to pain; no fractures, dislocations, or subluxations on cervical spine AP, lateral, open mouth, flexion extension, and oblique views. Cervical MRI: no disk herniation, spinal stenosis, or occult process.

Questions: What is the cause of this patient's neck pain and headaches? Which is the diagnostic procedure of choice to confirm the cause? Is there a specific procedure you would recommend for treatment?

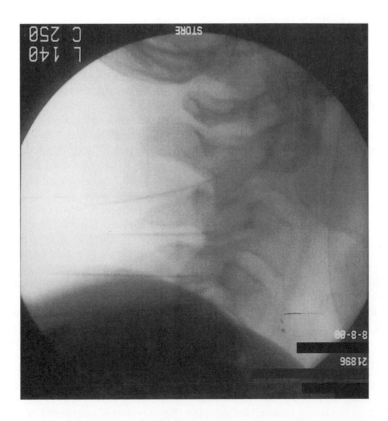

Answer: Cervical zygapophyseal joint syndrome resulting from hyperextension/hyperflexion injury of the cervical spine ("whiplash"). Medial branch block can confirm the cause. Radiofrequency ablation is the recommended treatment.

Discussion: Hyperextension-hyperflexion injury of the cervical spine—or "whiplash"—has been described in the medical literature for many years. The injury was first described in 1928 by orthopedist Harold Crowe. The incidence of chronic pain following motor vehicle accidents has been debated in the medical literature. Studies show that most patients who present with neck pain and other complaints related to whiplash injuries do improve; however, the residual group in whom symptoms persist beyond 6 months remain a significant clinical problem.

The injury tends to occur as a result of sudden deceleration (a front-end collision) or sudden acceleration (a rear-end collision). In motor vehicle accidents, the neck is subject to forces in flexion, extension, and lateral flexion, along with shear forces parallel to the direction of impact. There are many variables that dictate the severity and extent of cervical spine trauma in motor vehicle accidents: direction and amount of force, time of application of force, area of impact, speed of impact, position of structures at the time when force is applied, frequency with which the force is applied, and the strength of the involved structures. The forces applied to the cervical spine can result in subluxations, fractures, dislocations, spinal cord injury, strains, and sprains.

The **shear forces** that act on the cervical spine are perpendicular to the long access of the neck. The type of shear depends upon the direction of impact. In a front-impact collision/deceleration injury, the shear forces result in compression of the zygapophyseal joints and stretching of the capsular and annular fibers in the anterior part of the disk. In rear-impact collisions/acceleration injuries, the shear forces result in distraction of the facet joint, with stretching of the capsular and retrograde stretching of the annular disk fibers. In a rear-end/acceleration injury, the vehicle accelerates forward at the time of impact, and the occupant's head and neck is initially forced into flexion within 100–150 milliseconds. The time for cervical muscles to respond to sudden forces is believed to be almost 200 milliseconds. Thus the muscles that normally control the direction and amplitude of motion do not have time to respond to the forces being applied to them. This results in significant soft tissue damage, even in minor impact (at an impact speed of 3–5 miles per hour). After the initial flexion moment, about 100 milliseconds later, there is forced extension of the head and neck as the torso, induced by the car seat, travels anteriorly under the head.

Tissue injury has been evaluated by indirect means because most whiplash injuries are not fatal. Injuries to the facet joints include fractures of the joint itself and/or the supporting pillars. These areas are difficult to image on plain radiography. The disk can be avulsed from the end plate and annular tears can occur. Data from some studies suggest that the age-adjusted prevalence of degenerative changes is higher in patients who have sustained a whiplash injury, but data from other studies has shown no difference. Muscles in the anterior portion of the cervical spine can be partially or completely torn. Ligament injuries can include tears of the anterior longitudinal ligament as well as the alar ligament at the C1-2 complex. Damage to the posterior longitudinal ligament and ligamentum flavum is not usually caused by whiplash. If present, it reflects a higher degree of injury. Injury to the posterior elements (pedicles, lamina, facet joints, and transverse processes) can occur, but often cannot be diagnosed by routine imaging techniques and may require specialized testing, such as CT scanning and MRI.

Symptoms of whiplash injury are multiple and diversified. They may include pain in the shoulder and interscapular area, low back pain, occipital headaches, arm and hand numbness, vertigo, and auditory and visual disturbances. The neck pain is usually described as a dull or sharp aching, worse with movement and localized over the back of the neck; it is also associated with neck stiffness. Most patients who sustain whiplash injury have symptoms within the first 2 days of injury. Recovery is complete in 57% of patients. The recovery period is about 3 months, and the majority of patients reach their final stage within 1 year. The incidence of chronic neck pain is 14–42% in cases of whiplash injury. Poor prognostic indicators for recovery after whiplash injury are severity or duration of symptoms, age over 50 years, ongoing litigation, pain radiation into the upper extremities, and associated thoracic and lumbar pain.

The **cervical zygapophyseal joint** appears to be the primary pain generator in whiplash syndromes; one study found it to be the source of pain in 54% of patients after motor vehicle accidents. This joint has been studied in asymptomatic patients, and pain referral patterns have been generated. Randomized studies of intra-articular corticosteroid injections for chronic pain in the cervical zygapophseal joints revealed that less than 50% of patients reported pain relief of 1-week duration, and less than 20% reported relief of 1-month duration.

Intra-articular steroids are not effective in the treatment of zygapophyseal joint pain from whiplash.

Treatment of whiplash injury includes early mobilization; cervical collars have been shown to be unsuccessful in helping to relieve the pain from whiplash injuries. Treatment modalities could include analgesics, antidepressants, exercise, physical therapy, traction, heat, ice, manipulations, intra-articular injections, cervical pillows, transcutaneous electrical nerve stimulation, ultrasound, epidural, trigger point injections, muscle relaxants, and psychological interventions. Unfortunately, most of these therapeutic interventions lack scientific validity, and those that have been evaluated in a scientific manner show very little benefit. Whiplash-associated disorders have been classified by the Quebec Task Force in grades 0 to 4 based on the severity of injury.

Treatments are based upon the severity of the whiplash-associated disorder. Most patients with grade II injuries are treated with non-narcotic analgesics and nonsteroidal anti-inflammatories. In grade III injuries, narcotic analgesics may need to be prescribed for the acute phase.

Quebec Classification of Whiplash-Associated Disorders

Grade	Clinical Description
0	No neck complaint; no physical sign(s)
I	Complaint of neck pain, stiffness, or tenderness only; no physical sign(s)
II	Neck complaint and musculoskeletal sign(s)
III	Neck complaint and neurological sign(s)
IV	Neck complaint and fracture or dislocation

Recent studies have attempted to localize the source of pain to the zygapophyseal joint and the associated medial branch responsible for innervation. Radiofrequency ablation has been performed successfully using an extensive and meticulous approach, and some patients with chronic zygapophyseal joint injuries secondary to motor vehicle accidents have had relief.

Clinical Pearls

1. Cervical zygapophyseal joint injury is a diagnosis of exclusion when all other causes of neck pain have been eliminated.

2. Most patients with whiplash-associated disorder tend to reach maximal improvement within 1 year.

3. Of patients with whiplash injuries, 14–42% experience chronic neck pain.

4. Cervical medial branch block (see figure) and radiofrequency ablation may be of diagnostic and potential therapeutic benefit for patients with cervical zygapophyseal joint injury secondary to motor vehicle accidents.

5. Physical findings are localized by reproducing the pain with direct palpation over the posterior elements and with stressed extension and rotation.

REFERENCES

1. Barnsley L, Lord S, Bogduk N: Whiplash Injury. Pain 58:283–307,1994.
2. Barnsley L, Lord S, Wallis BJ, et al: Lack of the Effect of Intra-articular Corticosteroid for Chronic Pain in the Cervical Zygapophyseal Joints. New Engl J Med 330:1047–1050, 1994.
3. Barnsley L, Lord S, Wallis BJ, et al: The Prevalence of Zygapophyseal Joint Pain after Whiplash. Spine 20:20–26,1995.
4. Dwyer A, April C, Bogduk M: Cervical Zygapophyseal Joint Pain Patterns 1. A Study in Normal Volunteers. Spine 15:453–457, 1990.
5. Gruber R, Botwin K, Bouchlas C, Torres F: Pathophysiology of Spinal Trauma in Motor Vehicle Accidents. PM&R 12(1):39–72, 1998.
6. Holm HL: Soft Tissue Injuries of The Neck in Automobile Accidents: Factors Influencing Prognosis. J Bone Joint Surg 54A:1675–1682, 1974.
7. Schrader H: Natural Evolution of Late Whiplash Syndrome Outside Medical Legal Context. Lancet 347:127-133, 1996.
8. Spitzer WO, Skovron ML, Salmi LR, et al: Scientific Monograph of the Quebec Task Force on Whiplash Associated Disorders: Redefining "Whiplash" and its Management. Spine 20(suppl): 1S–73S, 1995.
9. Twomey L, Taylor JR: Whiplash Syndrome Pathology and Physical Treatment. J Manual Manipulative Therapy 1:26–29, 1993.

PATIENT 16

A 32-year-old woman with sudden onset of paraplegia and severe low back pain

A 32-year-old woman presents to the emergency department with a sudden onset of severe low back pain and paraplegia. She reports a history of increasing low back pain over the last several weeks. However, this morning when she got up and went to the bathroom, she felt severe burning pain in her low back. She then noted the rapid onset of numbness and weakness in her legs, initially the left, then the right, and then the numbness extended up the abdomen to just above the umbilicus. She was unable to move either leg and was transported to the emergency department by ambulance. The patient gives a history of being involved in a motor vehicle accident about 10 years ago and of subsequent problems with recurring back pain. She describes the previous, recurring pain as aching in nature and quite different from the present back pain. She has not taken any medication for the pain. She has not been able to urinate at home.

Physical Examination: Temperature 97.2°; pulse 62; respiration 24; blood pressure 117/69. Skin: normal. HEENT: normal. Chest: clear. Cardiac: normal. Abdomen: soft, with normal active bowel sounds. Musculoskeletal: normal range of motion in the upper and lower extremities; normal strength in the upper extremities; no voluntary movement in lower extremities. Neurologic: cranial nerves II–XII intact; 3+ knee jerks bilaterally; sustained clonus in both ankles; positive Hoffmann sign bilaterally; positive Babinski sign bilaterally; impaired light touch and pinprick sensation approximately below the T7–8 level bilaterally; absence of proprioception in both lower extremities. Rectal: no light touch, pinprick, and pressure sensation; no voluntary anal contraction; positive bulbocavernous reflex. Urologic: large amount of urine upon placement of Foley catheter.

Laboratory Findings: WBC 5500 /μl; hct 37.2%; platelets 197,000 /μl; Westergren ESR 9 mm/hr. Urinalysis: normal. Electrolytes: normal. VDRL nonreactive; HIV nonreactive; Lyme titer negative; ANA negative. CSF: WBC 7/ml; RBC 2/ml; monocytes 98%; glucose 91 mg/dl; protein 47 mg/dl; VDRL nonreactive; cryptococcal antigen negative; malignant cell negative. Blood culture: no growth. CSF culture: no growth. Spinal myelogram: mild posterior spondylosis present at C4–5, C5–6, and C6–7 without cord compression; small herniated nucleus pulps at the T6–7, T9–10, T11–12, and L5–S1 levels with no cord compression. Brain MRI: normal pre and post-contrast studies of the brain. Spinal MRI: degenerative vertebral discs at T6–7, T9–10, and T 11–12, and L5–S1; hemangioma at the T7 vertebral body; no canal stenosis; no cord compression.

Question: What is the cause of this patient's paraplegia?

Diagnosis: Acute transverse myelitis.

Discussion: Acute transverse myelitis (ATM) is a relatively uncommon clinical diagnosis. The disorder affects all age groups and does not discriminate according to gender. Conservative estimates of incidence is 1–5 per million population. It is characterized by initial back or radicular pain, followed by rapidly ascending paresthesias or sensory loss and motor weakness. **Bowel and bladder dysfunction** is a common presentation. The symptoms evolve within hours to several days, with maximum clinical signs 4 weeks after onset at latest. The back pain is described as sharp or pinching in the thoracic or lumbar area with sudden onset. Many patients describe a tight banding or girdle-like feeling around the trunk and a hypersensitivity to touch in that area. The paresthesia and leg weakness is an ascending form, which may or may not be symmetrical. The degree of severity varies between slight muscle weakness and total paralysis.

In about one-third of patients, acute transverse myelitis occurs in the setting of another illness. ATM is thought to be an inflammatory disorder of the spinal cord. Etiologically, it can be divided into four groups: **(1)** cellular autoimmune response triggered by infection or vaccination, sometimes called idiopathic ATM; **(2)** myelitis due to direct infection—usually viral—of the spinal cord; **(3)** myelitis in the context of systemic autoimmune disease, especially collagen disease such as SLE; **(4)** vascular insufficiency–induced nonspecific inflammation of a spinal cord segment, with concomitant loss of function.

The diagnosis of ATM is based on the clinical presentation and exclusion of the other cause of sudden-onset paraplegia, transverse myelopathy. It is important to rule out spinal cord compression due to an abscess, tumor, herniated intervertebral disc, or fracture. Spinal MRI, CSF findings, and some electrophysiologic studies have been used as tools to establish a proper diagnosis. **MRI study** has specific value to exclude spinal cord compression, but MRI findings in ATM are nonspecific and variable. T1-weighted images may reveal an enlargement of the spinal cord. On T2-weighted images, a diffuse hyperintensity of the affected spinal cord segment is sometimes noticed, which may reflect the inflammation, ischemia, and demyelination. Gadolinium has been used to enhance the lesion of the affected cord segment in MRI studies of ATM. Nearly 80% of lesions are found at the thoracic spinal cord region. This has been attributed to the relatively poor blood support to this region of spinal cord in comparison to the other levels of the spinal cord and brain.

CSF findings vary considerably in patients and in course of the disease. There are specific CSF changes in different etiological ATM cases. Most often there is moderate lymphocytic pleocytosis and an elevated protein level.

Electromyography and somatosensory evoked potential studies can be used to distinguish central versus peripheral nervous system damage for differential diagnosis.

The differential diagnosis includes multiple sclerosis (MS), Guillain-Barré syndrome, and spinal cord infarction. ATM can be an initial presentation of MS. In one study that reviewed clinical features of acute myelitis in 36 patients, 16 developed clinical definite MS during a 4.5-year follow-up period. Brain MRI is particularly important to distinguish ATM from MS. The finding of periventricular white matter lesions in ATM patients indicates that the risk of evolution to MS is as high as 90%. The ATM patients with a normal brain MRI carry an approximately 5% risk of late development of MS.

Treatments for ATM vary depending on etiology. For noninfectious ATM, corticosteriod therapy is generally recommended. The method and course of steroid administration are variable, usually from 1 week to 1 month. If patients are medically stable, rehabilitation therapy can be started to help with functional recovery and bowel and bladder management.

The outcome of ATM can be classified as good, fair, and poor. About 44% of patients have a good outcome: they have no residual signs and symptoms, or mild neurological abnormality and mildly disturbed micturition. Around 33% of the patients have a fair outcome: they are functional and ambulatory, but may have spastic paresis and prominent sphincter disturbance. The remaining patients have poor outcome, and if no improvement is seen by 3 months, significant recovery is unlikely. They have severe neurological deficits, are usually wheelchair-bound, and have no control of bowel and bladder. The predictors of a poor outcome are back pain as the first symptom, a very acute course with maximal symptoms reached within hours, spinal shock, and sensory impairments up to the level of cervical dermatomes.

In the present patient, image studies were very nonspecific. There was no spinal cord compression, and though some spondylosis and herniated nucleus pulposi were found, they were not severe enough to cause her paraplegia. She had severe low back pain as an initial symptom, with an acute course. The diagnosis was based on the history and physical exam. She was treated with Decadron and then Solu-Medrol for 10 days. However, little motor function was recovered, and she was transferred to a rehabilitation facility. The patient had regained some strength and sensation by the time of discharge from the rehabilitation hospital 1 month later, but she still could not stand or walk. Severe spasticity developed, requiring high doses of baclofen. The patient still needed in and out catheterization for bladder management and a bowel program for bowel management.

Clinical Pearls

1. Acute transverse myelitis is an inflammatory disorder of the spinal cord characterized by an acute onset of back pain, paresthesias, bilateral lower extremity weakness, and bowel and bladder dysfunction.

2. ATM can be etiologically divided into four groups: infection triggered autoimmune response; direct spinal cord infection; context of systemic autoimmune disease; and nonspecific inflammation of the spinal cord induced by vascular insufficiency.

3. ATM may be the initial presentation of multiple sclerosis (MS). The brain MRI is particularly important for distinguishing ATM from MS.

4. With the exception of infectious ATM, steroid therapy is the generally recommended treatment.

5. The outcome of ATM varies between total recovery and severe neurologic deficit.

REFERENCES

1. Jeffery DR, Mandler RN, Davis LE: Transverse myelitis: Retrospective analysis of 33 cases, with differentiation of cases associated with multiple sclerosis and parainfectious events. Arch Neurol 50:532, 1993.
2. Knebusch M, Strassburg HM, Reiners K: Acute transverse myelitis in childhood: Nine cases and review of the literature. Devel Med Child Neurol 40:631–639, 1998.
3. Rudick AR: Multiple sclerosis and related conditions. In Weksler BB (ed): Cecil Textbook of Medicine, 20th ed. Philadelphia, WB Saunders, 1996.
4. Thomas M, Thomas J Jr: Acute transverse myelitis. J Louisiana State Med Soc 149:75–77, 1997.

PATIENT 17

A 28-year-old man with right shoulder pain

A 28-year-old, right-handed man presents with diffuse right shoulder pain of 3- to 4-week duration. The pain started gradually and it is sharp and sometimes stabbing. Right shoulder movements are decreased. He also complains of pain in the interscapular region that radiates to the right arm and includes vague numbness. He does not have neck pain. He believes that his right arm has weakened. There is no history of trauma, viral illness, or surgery. He has no symptoms on the left. Past history is not significant for any prior musculoskeletal problems.

Physical Examination: General: height 6 feet, weight 165 pounds. Gait: no antalgia or spasticity. Musculoskeletal: no obvious deformity in right shoulder or cervical spine; decreased scapulothoracic rhythm on right; no scapular winging or atrophy; range of motion in right shoulder decreased in all directions, especially on external rotation (extremely painful); overall examination difficult due to marked guarding by patient; diffuse tenderness of right shoulder, especially in right periscapular region. Neurologic: deep tendon reflexes at biceps, triceps, and brachioradialis 2+ and symmetrical; light touch and pin- prick normal. Circulation: normal. Spurling's test: negative.

Laboratory Findings: X-rays of right shoulder and cervical spine: normal. Electrodiagnostic evaluation: normal median and ulnar motor and sensory nerve conductions; normal superficial radial sensory nerve conduction. Electromyography (EMG): normal biceps, deltoid, triceps, brachioradialis, pronator teres, first dorsal interosseous, and abductor pollices brevis muscles; cervical paraspinals also normal; mildly increased insertional activity of supraspinatus, but no spontaneous activity and interference decreased; increased insertional activity of infraspinatus, plus spontaneous activity of 3+ fibrillations and positive sharp waves. Note: only 1–2 fast-firing motor units activated at maximal effort.

Questions: What is your initial diagnosis? What additional diagnostic test(s) would you order?

Diagnosis: Right suprascapular focal neuropathy at the spinoglenoid notch.

Discussion: Focal neuropathy at the spinoglenoid notch is not very common, but it remains important in the differential diagnoses of rotator cuff structural problems, C5–6 radiculopathy, and upper trunk brachial plexopathy (Parsonage Turner syndrome). Causes of entrapment of the suprascapular nerve include traction or kinking of the nerve, close trauma, repetitive exercise, or compression by ganglion cyst. Certain sports such as volleyball have also been noted to be associated with the lesions. Patients usually have nonspecific pain, weakness, and atrophy of the spinatus musculature.

Several anatomic studies have been carried out. Entrapment by the inferior transverse scapular ligament, also termed the spinoglenoid ligament (SGL), has been suggested in those patients with no cystic or mass compression. During cross-body adduction and internal rotation of the glenohumeral joint, the interaction of the SGL and the posterior capsule results in a tightening of the SGL. The suprascapular nerve moves laterally and gets stretched underneath the SGL in this position. Men are more commonly affected than women. A cadaver study suggests that the SGL may be absent in 50% of females and 13% of males.

Clinical diagnosis is difficult unless patients have isolated infraspinatus atrophy with or without pain. Plain radiographs are normal in the majority of cases. Electromyography shows evidence of denervation in the infraspinatus and prolonged suprascapular motor latency on recording from the infraspinatus. Ultrasound, MRI, or magnetic resonance arthrography (MRA) is suggested to localize and characterize the presence of a mass compression. In addition, MRI may demonstrate atrophy of the spinatus muscles. MRA allows visualization of lesions of the glenoid labrum and in some cases, demonstrates cysts filling. Acute/subacute denervation is best seen on T2-weighted, fast-spin echo images with fat saturation, showing increased signal intensity related to neurogenic edema. Chronic denervation is best seen on T1-weighted, spin echo images, which demonstrate loss of muscle bulk and diffuse areas of increased signal intensity within the muscle.

In the absence of a well-defined lesion producing mechanical compression of the suprascapular nerve, suprascapular neuropathy may be treated nonoperatively. Stretching exercises for shoulder flexors and scapular stabilizers are recommended. When mechanical compression and infraspinatus atrophy are present, surgical treatment is recommended.

If there is a noncommunicating cyst compressing the nerve, sonographically guided aspiration is an effective and inexpensive—as well as less-invasive—method to treat these cysts. When surgical treatment is delayed and there is advanced muscle atrophy, the pain usually subsides after release of the suprascapular ligament but the atrophy persists in the majority of patients. If labral lesions are associated with the cyst, arthroscopy, repair of the lesions, and either arthroscopic debridement or direct open decompression and excision of the cyst are recommended.

In the present patient, physical examination was difficult. The provisional diagnosis was a rotator cuff tear in the right shoulder. However, EMGs were diagnostic for a distal suprascapular neuropathy. Due to his poor pain tolerance, suprascapular nerve conduction was not done. MRI of the spinoglenoid notch area, to rule out a cystic compression (see figure), did show a cyst with communication to the glenoid labrum. The patient has been referred for an arthroscopic repair of the labrum and an open decompression of the cyst.

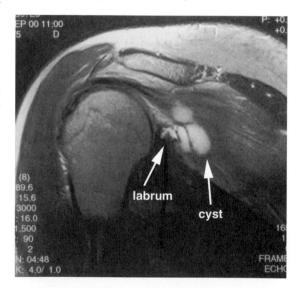

Clinical Pearls

1. About 50% of females lack an inferior transverse scapular ligament, also called the spinoglenoid ligament.

2. Ganglion cysts are the most common cause of suprascapular nerve compression at the spinoglenoid area.

3. Needle EMG of supraspinatus and infraspinatus should be a part of routine electrodiagnostic evaluation of patients with vague shoulder complaints.

4. Ultrasonographically guided aspiration of noncommunicating cysts is a useful and less-invasive method of treatment.

REFERENCES

1. Demirhan M, Imhoff AB, Debski RE, et al: The spinoglenoid ligament and its relationship to the suprascapular nerve. J Shoulder Elbow Surg 7: 238–243, 1998.
2. Martin SD, Warren RF, Martin TL, et al: Suprascapular neuropathy. Results of nonoperative treatment. J Bone Joint Surg Am 79:1159–1165, 1997.
3. Post M: Diagnosis and treatment of suprascapular nerve entrapment. Clin Orthop 368:92–100, 1999

PATIENT 18

A 37-year-old man with chronic right foot pain and temperature changes

A 37-year-old man sustained an injury to the dorsal aspect of his right foot when a 100-pound box fell from a height of approximately 4 feet. The patient experienced initial bruising and swelling, which resolved after 2 weeks. X-rays were negative for fracture. Treatment consisted of nonsteroidal anti-inflammatories (NSAIDs) and restricted weightbearing. Now, 2 months after the accident, he continues to complain of intermittent burning pain of the foot and toes, with purplish discoloration and coolness of the skin over the foot. The patient wants to know if his foot is going to eventually feel better, or if there is possible loss of blood supply.

Physical Examination: Skin: hyperhidrosis of right foot, with mottling erythema of distal foot and toes. Temperatures: right foot 28.9° C, left foot 33° C. Pulses: dorsalis pedis and posterior tibial 2+ and bounding. Musculoskeletal: active range of motion limited in metatarsophalangeal flexion of right great toe; normal dorsiflexion and plantar flexion at ankle mortis; normal eversion of subtalar motion, but limited inversion secondary to pain. Neurologic: tenderness (allodynia) over distal medial foot and along first metatarsal ray; 5/5 strength on knee extension, dorsiflexion, and plantar flexion bilaterally; normal pinprick; two-point discrimination with mild paraesthesia along medial border of first ray. Gait: normal toe and heel walking.

Laboratory Findings: CBC, ESR, ANA: normal. Electrolytes normal. Nerve conduction studies of tibial motor, peroneal motor, and sural sensory: normal.

Questions: What is the diagnosis? Which test(s) would be helpful in confirming the diagnosis?

Answers: Complex regional pain syndrome type I (CRPS). Scintigraphy (triple-phase bone scan) can be helpful.

Discussion: CRSP types I and II are names developed by a consensus group in 1993 to describe pain syndromes previously called reflex sympathetic dystrophy and causalgia. CRPS I describes a constellation of signs and symptoms that develop after an initiating noxious event, predominantly in the distal region of an extremity. It is not limited to the distribution of a single nerve and exceeds the expected clinical course of the inciting event. CRPS II represents burning pain that develops after specific nerve injury. In CRPS I, early signs and symptoms include warmth, edema of the extremity, abnormal pseudomotor activity, allodynia, and hyperpathia in the region of pain. Allodynia has been defined as the perception of pain elicited by a non-noxious stimulus. Hyperpathia refers to pain in which the threshold to initiate pain is raised, but once exceeded is more severe than expected. Cyanosis and mottling of the skin may be present in CRPS I, as well as a movement disorder characterized by difficulty initiating movement, weakness, tremor, spasm, and dystonia.

CRPS I or reflex sympathetic dystrophy (RSD) has three progressive stages if not treated. **Stage I** usually lasts approximately 3 months and includes the characteristics listed above. **Stage II** is often called the dystrophic phase, and can include more severe and diffuse pain, brawny edema, cooling of the extremity, neural changes, stiffness, and muscle wasting. After approximately 9 months, **stage III** begins, including irreversible muscle atrophy, pain involving the entire limb, flexor tendon contractures, and diffuse bone deossification.

Much controversy surrounds the etiology and pathophysiology of CRPS. Potential causes include local infection, fracture, peripheral neuropathy, myocardial infarction, chronic obstructive pulmonary disease, and strokes resulting in hemiplegia—although in many cases no cause is identified. The sympathetic nervous system produces **sympathetically maintained pain** (SMP) in CRPS when sympathetic reflexes to a noxious stimuli begin a positive feedback cycle in the spinal cord. Continuous activity and afferent nociceptive neurons can cause pain (allodynia and hyperalgesia) through sensitization of the dorsal horn neurons.

Note that the consensus group mentioned above reported SMP not as a requirement, but rather an *associated phenomenon* in CRPS. Therefore, CRPS can be diagnosed without the presence of sympathetically maintained pain. The **psychological aspects** of CRPS are not to be ignored. An abnormally high prevalence of psychopathology is seen in patients who have been diagnosed with the syndrome. It is often difficult to distinguish whether these psychological issues are the cause or the effect. Before diagnosis is made or treatment begins, it is important to have objective evidence of the presence of CRPS. Hysteria, malingering, somatization disorder, anxiety, and depression are commonly seen in patients with presumed CRPS.

Diagnosis remains a controversial issue and continues to be based on clinical findings. Three conditions considered by most doctors to reflect CRPS include: (**1**) burning, diffuse pain, with (**2**) loss of motor function, and (**3**) sympathetic dysfunction. Objective studies and procedures include plain radiographs, sympathetic blocks, resting skin temperatures, thermography, resting sweat output, isolated cold stress testing, and scintigraphy. A recent review by Fournier and Holder concluded that radionuclide bone scintigraphy (triple-phase bone scan) can provide objective evidence for the clinical entity called RSD. Especially in stage I patients, a high degree of sensitivity and specificity has been shown. In interpreting the triple-phase bone scan, diagnostic criteria for CRPS (reported by Holder and MacKinnon) include diffuse increased activity with increased flow on the angiogram, diffusely increased blood pool phase activity, and diffusely increased delayed activity in RSD. The delayed increased activity with juxta-articular accentuation seems to be the most sensitive finding supporting the diagnosis of CRPS.

In the present patient, triple-phase bone scan (*see figure*) revealed a diffuse area of increased uptake, which is characteristic of CRPS. He is in late stage I or early stage II CRPS.

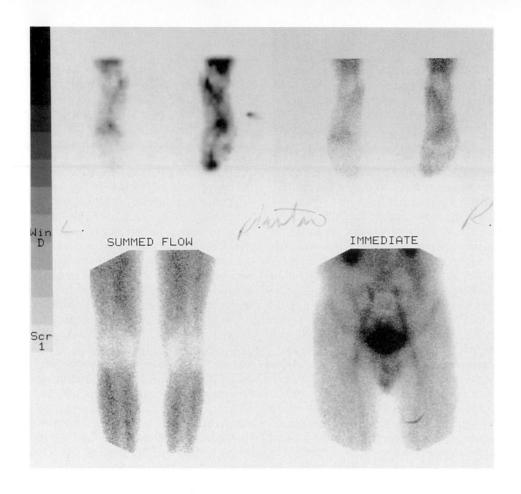

SUMMED FLOW   IMMEDIATE

Clinical Pearls

1. CRPS I (reflex sympathetic dystrophy) and II (causalgia) are new terms developed to describe pain syndromes.

2. Suspect CRPS I when symptoms include burning, swelling, and temperature fluctuation.

3. Be cautious to include objective findings in diagnosing CRPS. Not all unexplained pain is CRPS.

4. Triple-phase bone scan is an objective test that can be used to support the diagnosis. Sensitivity of the scan is inversely related to the duration of the symptoms.

5. Sympathetically maintained pain is an associated phenomenon, but not a requirement for the diagnosis of CRPS.

REFERENCES

1. Brown DL: Somatic Or Sympathetic Block For Reflex Sympathetic Dystrophy: Which Is Indicated. Hand Clinics 13(3): 485–497, 1997.
2. Fournier RS, Holder LE: Reflex Sympathetic Dystrophy: Diagnostic Controversies. Semin Nucl Med 28(1): 116–123, 1998.
3. Kasdan ML, Johnson AL: Reflex Sympathetic Dystrophy. Occup Med 13(3): 521–531, 1998.
4. Wilson PR: Posttraumatic Upper Extremity Reflex Sympathetic Dystrophy: Clinical Course, Staging, and Classification of Clinical Forms. Hand Clinics 13(3):367–372, 1997.

PATIENT 19

An 84-year-old man who sustained a fall

An 84-year-old man who resides in a nursing home was found by a nurse on the floor of his room. The nurse reportedly heard a "crashing noise," followed by a scream. The man was on his right side, with his lunch tray next to him and spilled food items nearby. He told the nurse that he fell as he was trying to go to the restroom. He denies any chest pain, shortness of breath, or altered motor control. He has a medical history of hypertension, peripheral vascular disease, and sinusitis. His medicines include dyazide, aspirin, and terfenadine, and zolpidem for sleep.

Physical Examination: Temperature 98°, pulse 110, respirations 20, blood pressure 110/67 mmHg. Skin: 3-cm contusion/abrasion on right elbow, small abrasion on right greater trochanter. HEENT: pupils equal and reactive to light and accomodation; normocephalic; oral cavity clear. Neurologic: alert and oriented to person, place, and situation; no focal neurologic deficits; normal gross visual acuity, including visual fields. Cardiac: increased rate, regular rhythm, no murmurs. Chest: clear. Abdomen: benign. Extremities: 1+ pretibial edema and venous insufficiency changes.

Laboratory Findings: WBC 7200/μl, Hct 32%, platelets 298,000/μl, blood sugar 74 mg/dl. BUN 52 mg/dl (normal 7–18), creatinine 1.9 mg/dl (0.7–1.3). Urinalysis: specific gravity 1.120 (normal 1.001–1.035), WBC 4/hpf, bacteria positive. Plain films of cervical spine, right elbow, and right hip: no acute abnormalities.

Questions: What is the most likely cause for the fall in this man? Give a differential diagnosis for possible reasons for falls in the elderly population.

Answers: Orthostatic hypotension secondary to dehydration in the setting of a urinary tract infection. See table for differential diagnosis.

Discussion: Falls occur in about one-third of community-dwelling individuals over the age of 65. The risk increases significantly in those older than 75. Of all fall-related deaths in the U.S., 70% occur among the elderly. Half of the people over 75 years old who fracture their hip from a fall die within 1 year of the injury.

While specific causes can result in a fall, the etiology is usually multifactorial. The risk of falling increases with the number of risk factors present. Some of the more common causes include impaired balance and motor control, sensory disturbance (touch and proprioception), slowed reaction time and righting reflex, prior fall, medications (especially sedatives, psychotropics, and antihypertensives used in combination), postural hypotension, visual impairments, vestibular disturbance, and psychological factors such as depression, inattention, and cognitive impairment. The common thread among all of these etiologies is that they are **intrinsic factors**: they relate directly to some physical or physiologic impairment.

Etiologies for Falls in the Elderly

- Neurologic: weakness, sensory impairment, poor motor planning, cognitive-behavioral
- Cardiovascular: orthostatic hypotension, dysrhythmia
- Prior fall
- Isolation
- Environmental factors: wet floor, poorly fitting shoes, obstacles
- Visual Impairments
- Vestibular impairment
- Gait disturbances / normal gait changes with aging

Extrinsic factors also account for falls in the elderly, but to a lesser extent. As we age, we are less able to adapt to our environment. Examples of extrinsic factors include inclement weather, loose rugs, physical barriers, poorly fitting shoes, and wet floors. While some studies cite use of an assistive device for ambulation as a risk factor for falls, it is not clear whether this is a result of the device itself, or due to the underlying gait disturbance in people who need assistive devices.

In the present patient, orthostatic hypotension developed because of dehydration from his urinary tract infection. Another factor is the underlying drop in cardiovascular regulatory control that occurs as we age; this is especially evident when the elderly move from sitting to standing. His antihypertensive medication certainly exacerbated the orthostatic hypotension, and the antihistamine could have caused some drowsiness. The patient was alone when he fell. This is a major risk factor because 95% of all falls in the geriatric population are unobserved.

Since many risk factors for falls cannot be altered (e.g., increasing age, neurologic impairment, sensory loss), our best hope for reducing the incidence of falls is by concentrating on the **reversible risk factors**. Examples include improving balance and motor control, reducing the number of medicines that can impair balance, behavioral intervention to improve planning and reduce impulsivity, and medical management to treat dehydration or illness. While some extrinsic factors pose a problem (poorly fitting shoes or wet floor), no studies find that physical barriers such as a room filled with furniture increase the risk of falls. Ironically, furniture may reduce the risk of falls in the elderly, because they may be familiar with the arrangement and use the pieces of furniture for stability while walking.

Clinical Pearls

1. Falls occur in approximately one in three community-dwelling people older than 65.
2. Ninety-five percent of falls in the elderly population are unobserved.
3. Falls in the elderly are usually multifactorial in etiology.
4. Intrinsic risk factors have a stronger role than extrinsic risk factors in the incidence of falls in the elderly population.
5. More than one-half of people over 75 who fracture a hip from a fall die within 1 year of the injury.

REFERENCES

1. Gill TM: Preventing Falls: To Modify the Environment or the Individual? J Am Geriatr Soc 47(12): 1471–1472, 1999.
2. Kiely DK, Kiel DP, Burrows AB, Lipsitz LA: Identifying Nursing Home Residents at Risk for Falling. J Am Geriatr Soc 46(5): 551–555, 1998.
3. Leipzig RM, Cumming RG, Tinetti ME: Drugs and Falls in Older People: A Systematic Review and Meta-Analysis: II. Cardiac and Analgesic Drugs. J Am Geriatr Soc 47(1): 40–50, 1999.
4. Means KM, Rodell DE, O'Sullivan PS: Obstacle Course Performance and Risk of Falling in Community-Dwelling Elderly Persons. Arch Phys Med Rehabil 79:1570–1576, 1998.
5. Pullen R, Heikaus C, Fusgen I: Falls of Geriatric Patients at the Hospital. J Am Geriatr Soc 47(12): 1481, 1999.
6. Rawsky E: Review of Literature on Falls Among the Elderly. Image J Nurs Scholar 30(1): 47–52, 1998.
7. Tinetti ME, Baker DI, McAvay G, et al: A Multifactorial Intervention to Reduce the Risk of Falling Among Elderly People Living in the Community. New Engl J Med 331(13): 821–827, 1994.

PATIENT 20

A 42-year-old man with groin and testicular pain after surgery

A 42-year-old man complains of groin and testicular pain following inguinal herniorrhaphy. He describes the pain as "burning, with pins and needles" and almost continuous. Little relief is obtained upon changing positions; performing a Valsalva maneuver; applying ice; resting; taking nonsteroidal anti-inflammatory drugs, gabapentin, dilantin, or tizanidine; or applying topical analgesics. He states that the pain has not eased in over 4 months since surgery, and that the only relief occurred when he received a "shot of something in the groin area." Relief was only short-lived, but nearly complete for 2–3 days. The patient denies night pain, sweats, weight-loss, fever, and rashes. He admits to decreased libido, which he attributes to chronic pain. He also denies pain in any other limb, as well as referral of pain to other areas of the body.

Physical Examination: General: appearance normal; no distress. Blood pressure 120/80, pulse 70, respirations 20. Chest: symmetric, clear. Cardiac: normal rate, rhythm; no murmurs. Abdomen: surgical scars consistent with history of inguinal herniorrhaphy; round, soft, nontender; no masses or organomegaly; normal bowel sounds. Extremities: normal. Neurologic: decreased sensitivity to light touch and pin prick in right groin area just adjacent to scrotum; also in lower right portion of scrotum; bulbocavernosus reflex intact. Rectal: normal.

Laboratory Findings: Blood count, serum electrolytes, sedimentation rate: normal. EMG: both lower limbs and lumbar paraspinal muscles normal.

Questions: Which nerve is involved in this patient's pain complaints? What procedure would be of most benefit?

Answers: The ilioinguinal nerve. Ilioinguinal nerve block would be of most benefit to this patient.

Discussion: This case illustrates **genitofemoral neuralgia**, a syndrome characterized by chronic pain and paresthesia in the region of genitofemoral nerve distribution. In women, chronic pain and tenderness in the groin, labia majora, and medial thigh can be caused by neuropathy of the genitofemoral nerve. Genitofemoral nerve entrapment has been described after inguinal herniorrhaphy, appendectomy, and cesarean section.

Obtain a careful history from patients with persistent pain and paresthesia in the inguinal region following surgery, and conduct the physical examination in conjunction with selected use of an **ilioinguinal-iliohypogastric nerve block** to confirm the diagnosis of nerve entrapment. Most patients with nerve entrapment experience complete relief of symptoms following serial injections, and require no further treatment. The remainder experience only temporary relief and require surgical interruption of the nerve involved. In those patients who obtain no relief from the nerve block, further work-up for a source of their pain is warranted.

The differential diagnosis of pain suggestive of genitofemoral or ilioinguinal neuralgia includes lesions (metastatic or infectious) in the lumbar plexus, or more proximally at the L1 nerve root (L1 radiculopathy). Thus, the EMG exam may be helpful in delineating more proximal sources of pain. Sippo and Gomez found, in a series of cases in which nerve blocks resulted in only temporary relief, that most patients had a subclinical recurrence of an inguinal hernia. Therefore, surgical consultation is recommended early in the work-up for patients presenting with groin and testicular (or labia majora) pain.

Other treatment includes paravertebral block of L-1 and L-2, or, in some recalcitrant cases, selective rhizotomies or neurectomy of the involved nerve. Neurectomy of the genitofemoral nerve proximal to the entrapment controlled the persistent pain in 10 of 13 patients with otherwise intractable pain.

Ilioinguinal nerve block is a relatively simple procedure that can offer dramatic relief for patients with complaints similar to those the present patient experienced. After confirmation of the correct injection site with a preceding dose of 2% lidocaine, neurolysis may be achieved by using a small (0.25 cc) amount of diluted phenol. The major side-effect of ilioinguinal nerve block is post-injection ecchymosis and hematoma. This side-effect can be avoided by immediate postblock pressure applied to the injection site. However, if the needle punctures the peritoneal cavity, colonic perforation and peritonitis may result. Accordingly, the clinician must proceed with caution to avoid such complications when attempting this block.

Clinical Pearls

1. Consider recurrence of an inguinal hernia in patients with post-herniorrhaphy–associated genitofemoral neuralgia.

2. An ilioinguinal-iliohypogastric nerve block will confirm the diagnosis of nerve entrapment in patients with genitofemoral neuralgia.

REFERENCES

1. Laha RK, Rao S, Pidgeon CN, Dujovny M: Genitofemoral neuralgia. Surg Neurol 8:280–282, 1977.
2. Perry CP: Laparoscopic treatment of genitofemoral neuralgia. J Am Assoc Gynecol Laparosc 4:231–234, 1997.
3. Schliack H, Schramm J, Neidhardt J: Selective rhizotomies for spinal root pain and neuralgia of the inguinal region. J Neurol 233:115–117, 1986.
4. Sippo WC, Gomez AC: Nerve-entrapment syndromes from lower abdominal surgery. J Fam Pract 25:585–587, 1987.
5. Starling JR, Harms BA, Schroeder ME, Eichman PL: Diagnosis and treatment of genitofemoral and ilioinguinal entrapment neuralgia. Surgery 102:581–586, 1987.
6. Wantz GE: Testicular atrophy and chronic residual neuralgia as risks of inguinal hernioplasty. Surg Clin North Am 73:571–581, 1993.

PATIENT 21

A 34-year-old woman with slurred speech and "droopy" eyelids

A 34-year-old woman presents with noticeable slurring of her words. The problem began 1 month ago, and worsens each day as the day progresses. She has been told that her eyelids appear "droopy." She reports that her arms tire easily with such activities as washing her hair. She has a history of breathing difficulty secondary to asthma, but believes she has been experiencing shortness of breath apart from that associated with asthma.

Physical Examination: Ophthalmologic: bilateral mild ptosis and weakness of eyelid closure; on routine testing, eye movements normal; with prolonged upward gaze, right eye drifted downward, and double vision occurred. Throat: tongue movement strong; voice quality normal. Neurologic: normal strength of all extremity muscle; mild weakening of finger extensors on repetitive testing; deep tendon reflexes 2+ and symmetric; sensation perception normal. Musculoskeletal: no apparent loss of muscle bulk; strength of neck flexors 4/5, extensors 5/5.

Laboratory Findings: Routine nerve conduction studies: normal. Repetitive nerve stimulation (of right radial nerve, recording over finger extensors): see figure; similar results found in right facial nerve, recording over nasalis. EMG (single fiber): increased jitter with blocking in right extensor digitorum communis and frontalis.

Question: What is the diagnosis?

Repetitive stimulation of radial nerve at rest

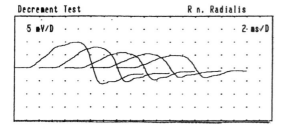

Repetitive stimulation of radial nerve 1 minute after exercise

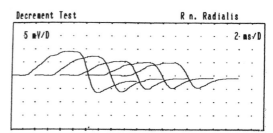

Repetitive stimulation of radial nerve immediately post-exercise

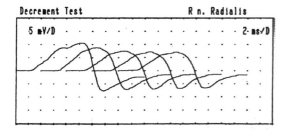

Repetitive stimulation of radial nerve 3 minutes after exercise

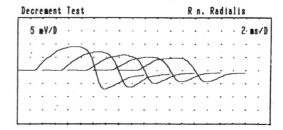

Diagnosis: Myasthenia gravis

Discussion: Repetitive nerve stimulation (RNS) is performed when a defect in neuromuscular transmission is suspected. In this patient, the symptoms and findings on exam suggested myasthenia gravis, a post-synaptic defect of neuromuscular transmission. Testing of selected nerve/muscle combinations offers the best chance for diagnostic results when there is muscle weakness. Accuracy of results is enhanced by choosing those muscles in which the examiner can control the movement. In evaluating for myasthenia gravis, use of the proximal nerves such as the radial, spinal accessory, and facial nerves is recommended.

First, the nerve is stimulated with the muscle at rest; then a series of stimulations (a minimum of four and a maximum of ten) is delivered. Subsequently, the muscle is exercised for 1 minute. If a significant decrement in the amplitudes is found at rest and immediately after exercise, RNS is repeated to determine if there has been an improvement (lessening) in the decrement. This improvement in the amplitudes is known as "repair" and is related to post-activation facilitation. When RNS is repeated 1 minute and 3 minutes after exercise, a comparative worsening of the decrement is found after 3 minutes because of post-activation exhaustion. The literature suggests that a decrement in amplitude greater than 10–12% is considered abnormal. This abnormal decrement should be found in at least two muscles.

Movement artifact from inadequate immobilization and submaximal stimulation can produce false positive results. If there is any question of the validity, the decrement should be reproduced on subsequent testing. The largest change in decrement amplitude is typically between the first and second response. The smallest compound muscle action potential amplitude is usually the fourth or fifth response. Following this, "recovery" occurs, and the amplitude levels out or increases to near its baseline value.

When the diagnosis of myasthenia gravis is suspected, but RNS failed to show a significant decremental response, single-fiber EMG (SFEMG) should be performed. In this test, a concentric needle electrode with a very small recording surface area (25 microns) is used to measure action potentials from individual muscle fibers innervated by the same motor units. The variation in the time interval between the pairs of muscle fibers is **neuromuscular jitter**, expressed in microseconds. Jitter is expressed as either mean consecutive difference or mean sorted difference. Jitter is considered abnormal if either the mean jitter from 20 muscle fiber pairs is greater than the upper limit of normal for the muscle being studied, or at least 10% of the pairs have jitter that is greater than the normal for a pair in that muscle. The extensor digitorum communis muscle is frequently studied in SFEMG. In generalized myasthenia gravis, increased jitter is found in this muscle nearly 90% of the time. The details of SFEMG are beyond the scope of this case, and references are provided for the interested reader.

Clinical Pearls

1. Both repetitive nerve stimulation and SFEMG may be abnormal with diseases (including ALS and polyneuropathies) other than those involving the neuromuscular junction. Thus, test results must be consistent with the clinical picture.

2. In pre-synaptic diseases (Lambert Eaton myathenic syndrome, botulism), there is a decrement at slow rates but an increment at fast rates of stimulation. Additionally, baseline CMAP amplitudes in these diseases are almost always abnormal.

3. Cooling of the muscle or the use of anticholinesterase medications may produce false negative results from these studies.

REFERENCES
1. Jablecki CK: AAEM Minimonograph #3: Myasthenia gravis. Muscle Nerve 14:391–397, 1991.
2. Keesey JC: AAEM Minimonograph #33: Electrodiagnositic approach to defects of neuromuscular transmission. Muscle Nerve 12:613–626, 1989.
3. Maselli RA: Electrodiagnosis of disorders of neuromuscular transmission. Ann NY Acad Sci 841:696–711, 1998.
4. Sanders DB, Howard JF: AAEE Minimonograph #25: Single fiber electromyography in myasthenia gravis. Muscle Nerve 9:809–819, 1986.

PATIENT 22

A 61-year-old man with a history of subarachnoid hemorrhage and decreasing participation in therapy

A 61-year-old man suffered a subarachnoid hemorrhage in the right frontal lobe after a fall off a horse. A craniotomy was done to evacuate the hemorrhage. He did well postoperatively, but had residual deficits in cognition and balance. He was initially lethargic, but showed gradual improvement and was at a Rancho los Amigos level 5 on the seventh postoperative day. His past history is significant only for depression. After 3 weeks of progress in rehabilitation, he shows decreasing participation in his therapies.

Physical Examination: Blood pressure 170/90, pulse 86, respiration 19, temperature 99°. General: not in acute cardiorespiratory distress. HEENT, heart, lungs, abdomen, and extremities: normal. Neurologic: awake; flat affect; nonverbal; no eye contact; sensation intact. Musculoskeletal: purposeful and localizing movements of upper extremities, but would not follow commands to cooperate with manual muscle testing; muscle stretch reflexes increased on left side.

Laboratory Findings: WBC 10,000/μl, Hct 48%, platelets 210,000/μl. Na$^+$ 140 mEq/L, K$^+$ 4.8 mEq/L. BUN 19 mg/dl, creatinine 1.1 mg/dl, calcium 9.5 mg/dl. Head CT (see figure): flattening of cortical sulci, periventricular lucency, and uniform ventricular dilatation

Question: What is the cause of the patient's deterioration?

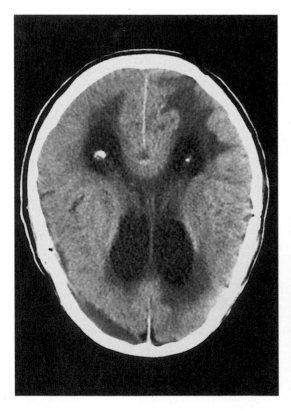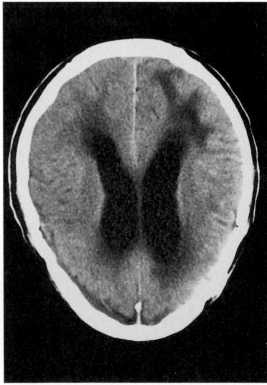

Diagnosis: Post-traumatic hydrocephalus

Discussion: Hydrocephalus is caused by a disruption in the normal flow and/or absorption of cerebrospinal fluid (CSF) through the ventricular system. Post-traumatic hydrocephalus is often of the normal pressure or communicating type, and is thought to be secondary to arachnoiditis and impaired resorption of CSF through the arachnoid granulations. The classic triad of dementia, incontinence, and gait ataxia is often described. However, this triad is not useful when dealing with severely brain-injured patients. Suspect post-traumatic hydrocephalus if the patient shows new-onset hypertension, failure to improve, or deterioration in cognition or behavior.

In a recent study, Marmarou et al. found that post-traumatic hydrocephalus developed in approximately 20% of 75 patients with severe traumatic brain injury, and ventriculomegaly developed in 44%. The diagnoses were arrived at via cerebrospinal fluid dynamics. Post-traumatic hydrocephalus should be differentiated from ventricular dilatation due to encephalomalacia. In encephalomalacia, ventriculomegaly is due to actual loss of brain tissue from atrophy or focal infarction from the brain injury, rather than to hydrocephalus itself.

Brain CT scans showing flattening of the cortical sulci, periventricular lucency, and uniform ventricular dilatation (as in the present patient) favor the diagnosis of post-traumatic hydrocephalus.

The treatment for post-traumatic hydrocephalus is placement of an extracranial shunt. In patients with a noncommunicating type, neuroendoscopic ventriculostomy may be considered as an alternative form of treatment.

Clinical Pearls

1. The classic triad of incontinence, gait ataxia, and dementia may not be useful for diagnosing post-traumatic hydrocephalus (PTH) in the brain-injured population. Deterioration in functional or neurological status may be the only indication that a patient has PTH.

2. PTH is often of the communicating (normal pressure) type.

3. Ventriculomegaly from PTH is differentiated from encephalomalacia by flattening of the cortical sulci, periventricular lucency, and uniform ventricular dilatation on CT scan.

4. The diagnosis of PTH is important since it is one of the few potentially treatable causes of neurological dysfunction after a TBI.

REFERENCES

1. Marmarou A, Foda MAA, Bandoh K, et al: Post-traumatic ventriculomegaly: hydrocephalus or atrophy? A new approach for diagnosis using CSF dynamics. J Neurosurg 85:1026–1035, 1996
2. O'Dell MW, Bell, KR, Sandel, ME: Brain injury rehabilitation. 2. Medical rehabilitation of brain injury. Arch Phys Med Rehabil 79 (suppl) 1:S10–S15, 1998.
3. Rosenthal M, Griffith ER, Kreutzer JS, Pentland B (eds): Rehabilitation of the Adult and Child with Traumatic Brain Injury, 3rd ed. Philadelphia, FA Davis, 1999.

PATIENT 23

A 2-year-old boy with poor muscle tone

A 2-year-old child is brought to your office by his parents for a routine habilitation clinic visit. He was born at term weighing 2730 g and suffered immediate distress, demonstrating poor muscle tone including total head lag and bilateral clubfoot deformity. He required resuscitation and oxygen, and received tube feedings for the first few months of life. Clubfoot surgery (posteromedial and tendo Achilles release) was performed at 9 months of age. A variety of diagnoses appear in his limited available records, including "talipes NOS," "lack norm physiol devel," "contracture of tendon," and a few GI and reflux-related ones.

At about 1 year of age, a videofluoroscopic swallowing study showed that the oral phase was severely impaired, and he still had difficulty extracting liquid from a bottle and collecting and propelling a paste-consistency bolus due to reduced lingual strength and coordination. He frequently lost control of the bolus prematurely and allowed it to fall into the pharynx. This resulted in increased oral transit time and residue in the oral cavity. The pharyngeal swallow was delayed 1–4 seconds, and he had vallecular and pyriform pooling. Laryngeal function was only mildly impaired, and aspiration was not observed. He continued to take a 27-calorie-per-ounce formula and baby foods, but weighed only 6.54 kg at 21 months of age; therefore, a gastrostomy tube was placed. He has received physical, occupational, and speech therapies through an early intervention program.

Physical Examination: General: thin appearing; weight 8.7 kg; facies unusual (see figure). Musculoskeletal: weight bears poorly when held in standing position. Gastrointestinal: gastrostomy in good condition. Abdomen: no mass, no organomegaly. Neurological: very poor muscle tone and head control; trunk control absent; supported sitting posture kyphotic; deep tendon reflexes not obtainable. Patient unable to move arms and legs against gravity. Sensation grossly intact. Extremities: some recurrence of equinovarus deformity, though partially rangeable; hips clinically not subluxable; no scoliosis; other range of motion actually excessive.

Laboratory Findings: Na^+ 139 mEq/L, K^+ 4.5 mEq/L, Cl^- 107 mEq/L. CO_2 24 mmol/L. Glucose 72 mg/dl, BUN 7 mg/dl, creatinine 0.2 mg/dl, phosphorus 6.3 mg/dl, albumin 3.5 g/dl, alkaline phosphatase 193 IU/L, triglyceride 52 mg/dl, magnesium 2 mg/dl (normal 2.1–2.9), T4 15.9, TSH 0.1, free T4 1.2, cortisol 3.7, and growth hormone 1.2.

Question: What is the diagnosis ?

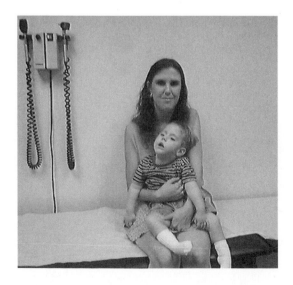

Diagnosis: Myotonic dystrophy, also known as Steinert's disease.

Discussion: Myotonic dystrophy is a very different disease for adults than for those with congenital onset. The child in this case has the classic "carp mouth" or myopathic facies that also appears in some other severe muscular disorders of a congenital nature, such as nemaline or central core. The mother of the present patient is also affected. A classic method of diagnosis is to shake hands with the mother and see if she has trouble releasing her grip, but this is not totally reliable. A slightly more sensitive method is to look for percussion myotonia of the thenar eminence, and DNA studies specific for this condition can also be ordered.

Myotonic dystrophy is an autosomal dominant disease caused by unstable expansion of the CTG repeats in the q13.3 band on chromosome 19, which encodes a protein kinase. The severity of the condition increases with each generation as the number of trinucleotide repeats increases. This mechanism is also behind several other dominantly inherited conditions, such as Huntington's disease, Machado-Joseph disease, fragile X syndrome, the olivopontocerebellar atrophies, and Friedreich's ataxia. The phenomenon of worsening and earlier onset in subsequent generations has been referred to as "genetic anticipation."

Some adults are unaware they have the condition; thus, it is wise to find out discreetly if they already know, even if they look just like this patient's mother. Individuals can be shocked and emotionally devastated to suddenly learn about it in too casual a manner. In some cases, the affected parent is truly undiagnosed and unaware, which is not at all uncommon in adult-onset cases of this disorder.

This particular child was actually diagnosed before he left the neonatal intensive care unit, as his mother's condition was known, and she is seen regularly through the adult Muscular Dystrophy Association clinic. (No one had yet used the term "myotonic disorders" as the primary diagnosis for their visits.) The mother receives regular EKGs for cardiac conduction deficits (cardiomyopathy) and ophthalmologic exams for cataracts as appropriate. She uses hinged ankle-foot orthotics because of distal weakness. Like most affected adults, she has a little myotonia, but does not find it a serious problem. EMG may not reveal myotonia in congenital cases for several years, but does reveal a myopathic pattern.

Males with myotonic dystrophy have reduced fertility as well as the classic hairline (frontal balding) and temporal wasting. In adults, intelligence is near normal or mildly affected. Children routinely have serious developmental delays and mental retardation or learning disability. They are prone to scoliosis; this patient's clubfoot is not at all uncommon. The most severely affected children not only have feeding problems, but also early ventilatory failure and problems handling secretions, which can lead to a significantly shortened lifespan. Creatine phosphokinase is normal or minimally elevated and therefore is not a helpful test.

The present patient is obviously weak rather than just hypotonic. Children who have hypotonia based on cerebral or metabolic conditions might have excess range of motion, but would require much less support, and could likely be enticed to show ability to reach overhead. With or without a family history, neuromuscular disease is clearly the diagnostic grouping to pursue in this case.

Clinical Pearls

1. Recent advances have changed our understanding of genetic transmission. The physician should stay abreast of genetic discoveries and know about specific disorders that present differently in children than adults.

2. A relatively "safe" swallow from the standpoint of aspiration risk does not guarantee adequate nutritional status.

3. The primary diagnostic factor in cases of congenital hypotonia is the presence or absence of weakness; sensory, bowel, and bladder abnormalities are a secondary factor and would indicate spinal cord dysfunction.

REFERENCES

1. Bodensteiner JB, Byler DL, Jaynes ME: The utility of the determination of CTG trinucleotide repeat length in hypotonic infants. Semin Pediatr Neurol 6(3):243–245; discussion 245–246, 1999.
2. Faulkner CL, Kingston HM: Knowledge, views, and experience of 25 women with myotonic dystrophy. J Med Genet 35(12):1020–1025, 1998.
3. Gennarelli M, Novelli G, Andreasi Bassi F, et al: Prediction of myotonic dystrophy clinical severity based on the number of intragenic CTG trinucleotide repeats. Am J Med Genet 65(4):342–347, 1996.
4. Lee SY, Chan KY, Chow CB: Survival of a 30-week baby with congenital myotonic dystrophy initially ventilated for 55 days. J Paediatr Child Health 35(3):313–314, 1999.
5. Takahashi S, Miyamoto A, Oki J, Okuno A: CTG trinucleotide repeat length and clinical expression in a family with myotonic dystrophy. Brain Dev 18(2):127–130, 1996.
6. Tanaka Y, Suzuki Y, Shimozawa N, et al: Congenital myotonic dystrophy: Report of paternal transmission. Brain Dev 22(2):132–134, 2000.
7. Tsuji S: Molecular genetics of triplet repeats: Unstable expansion of triplet repeats as a new mechanism for neurodegenerative diseases. Intern Med 36(1):3–8, 1997.

PATIENT 24

A 16-year-old girl with paraplegia after a fall

A 16-year-old, healthy girl was attempting to perform a cheerleader jump with her male partner at the local high school. When running in preparation of jumping up on her partner's shoulders, she slipped and fell on her upper back and neck. She developed immediate weakness and loss of sensation in her lower extremities. She presents to the local hospital's emergency department with paraplegia. A Foley catheter reveals residual urine of 600 cc. She gives no history of recent illness or fever. She has a past history bulimia and depression. Her mother reports that in the past the girl has made several suicide attempts. She was started on Solu-Medrol per the spinal cord injury steroid protocol.

Physical Examination: Temperature 98.3°; pulse 73; respirations 18; blood pressure 132/79. HEENT: normal. Chest: normal. Cardiac: normal. Abdomen: nontender; normal active bowel sounds. Musculoskeletal: full range of motion of upper and lower extremities and spine. Skin: normal. Neurologic: normal muscle tone and normal muscle stretch reflexes of upper and lower extremities; 0/5 strength in bilateral lower extremities; normal strength in bilateral upper extremities; absent sensation to pinprick and light touch 2 cm below the umbilicus, and bilaterally into both legs. Rectal: weak voluntary anal sphincter contraction; deep pressure sensation present, but absent pin prick and light touch.

Laboratory Findings: CBC, chemistries, and ESR: normal. Radiographs: C-spine normal; T-spine normal; L-spine normal. MRI of spine T10–L2: normal.

Question: What is the diagnosis?

Diagnosis: Conversion disorder with paraplegia.

Discussion: Conversion disorder is a subconscious functional deficit not attributable to organic disease. It is a manifestation of hysteria and is defined by the Diagnostic and Statistical Manual of Mental Disorders, 4th ed. (DSM-IV) as the following: ". . . an alteration or loss of physical functioning that suggests physical disorder, but that instead is apparently an expression of a psychological conflict or need." This is clearly separated from malingering, which is a conscious or intentionally produced loss of physical function for personal gain. In cases where the symptoms are difficult to explain neuroanatomically or are functionally inconsistent, hysteria should be part of the differential diagnosis.

The prevalence of conversion disorder may be as high as 2%, but it is difficult to study because of lack of agreement on the definition. Stefansson et al. reported an annual incidence of 11–22 per 100,000. The most common symptoms for patients diagnosed with conversion disorder are neurologic, followed by gastrointestinal. The most common specific neurologic complaint is "fits" (24%), followed by paralysis (10%) and "lump in the throat" (8%). Dickson et al. diagnosed 9.8% of new patients admitted to a spinal injury unit over a 1-year period with a conversion disorder.

Treatment of conversion disorders is variable. Watanabe et al. reviewed the literature regarding treatment for conversion disorder. The treatments consisted of physical therapy with exercise and electrical stimulation; psychiatric intervention with behavioral management, biofeedback, and Thiopentone; and a functional-based rehabilitation program. Watanabe suggested conventional rehabilitation therapy facilitated by behavioral modification and psychosocial support. Recovery can be expected within a few weeks in acute cases, but chronic conversion disorder can develop and symptoms may persist for up to 2 years. If patients do not improve with this program, it is reasonable to consider other etiologies such as an unresolved psychosocial stressor or perhaps a missed organic etiology. In one study it was estimated that 20–30% of individuals with a diagnosis of conversion disorder might have a missed organic lesion.

The present patient was paraplegic on discharge. However, 1 week after discharge her mother called the office and reported that her daughter was standing at her bedside, and she did not know what to do. She was told that this was a good sign of progressive neurologic recovery and to continue with the physical therapy program at school. In 3 months, the patient was ambulating and had returned to normal school activities, except with the limitation of avoiding any contact sports and cheerleading activities for the rest of the semester.

Clinical Pearls

1. In cases with a neurologic deficit that is difficult to explain by mechanism of injury or is functionally inconsistent, consider a differential diagnosis of conversion disorder.
2. Treatment consists of rehabilitation and psychiatric intervention.
3. Recovery usually is rapid and can be expected within a few weeks of "injury."
4. If recovery is not as expected, further work-up is required for a missed organic etiology or unresolved pyschosocial stressors.

REFERENCES

1. American Psychiatric Association: Diagnostic and Statistical Manual of Mental Disorders, 4th ed. Washington DC, American Pshychiatric Association, 1994.
2. Arkonac O, Guze SB: A family study of hysteria. N Engl J Med 268:238–242, 1963.
3. Dickson H, Cole A, Engel S, Jones R: Conversion reaction presenting as acute spinal cord injury. Med J Australia 141(7):427–429, 1984.
4. Stefansson J, Messina JA, Meyerwitz A: Hysterical neurosis, conversion type: Clinical and epidemiological considerations. Acta Psychitr Scand 84:288–293, 1976.
5. Teasell R, Shapira A: Chronic conversion disorders (letter). Arch Phys Med Rehabil 79:1483–1484, 1998.
6. Tomasson K, Kent D, Coryell W: Somatization and conversion disorders: Comorbidity and demographics at presentation. Acta Psychiatr Scand 84:288–293, 1991.
7. Watanabe TK, O'Dell MW, Togliatti TJ: Diagnosis and rehabilitation strategies for patients with hysterical hemiparesis: A report of four cases. Arch Phys Med Rehabil 79:709–714, 1988.
8. Withrington RH, Wynn Parry CB: Rehabilitation of conversion paralysis. J Bone Joint Surg Br 67B:635–637, 1985.

PATIENT 25

A 39-year-old man with low back and buttock pain

A 39-year-old man presents with a 10-week history of low back and bilateral proximal buttock pain. He had been doing yard work when the pain began. The patient has had difficulty with rotational and bending movement of his trunk since. He denies any numbness or tingling in the lower extremities. He has had no other trauma or injuries in the past. History reveals that he has had no recent fevers, night sweats, or bowel or bladder incontinence. The patient reports only 30–40% relief of his symptoms with a physical therapy program consisting of flexion exercises along with anti-inflammatories and analgesics.

Physical Examination: Vital signs: normal. Neurologic: motor exam 5/5 throughout upper and lower extremities; sensory intact to light touch, pinprick, and proprioception; reflexes symmetric and normoreflexic bilaterally; long tract signs negative. Musculoskeletal: tenderness in lumbar paraspinal area; no pain in back or legs on straight leg raising; pain reproduced with extension and rotation of lumbar trunk; lumbar flexion full and painless.

Laboratory Findings: Lumbosacral spine x-rays: no fractures, dislocations, or subluxations; mild sclerosis involving L4-5 and L5-S1 zygapophyseal joints.

Questions: What is the cause of this patient's low back pain? Which is the diagnostic procedure of choice for confirmation? Is there a treatment you would recommend for this condition?

Answers: Lumbar zygapophyseal (facet) joint syndrome. Medial branch block can confirm. Radiofrequency ablation can help in treatment.

Discussion: The **lumbar zagapophyseal (facet) joint** has been long considered a significant source of low back pain. Goldthwait stated in 1911 that "peculiarities of the facet joints" were responsible for low back pain and instability. Putti published an article in 1927 that reinforced Goldthwait's beliefs. It was Ghormeley who coined the term "facet joint syndrome" in 1933. He asserted: "To anyone who studies the skeleton, the vertebral peculiarities and their anatomy, the importance of the articular facet must be obvious." The mapping of pain responses after injections to local irritants was then expanded to include the lumbar zygapophyseal joints by Hirsch and colleagues. Corticosteroid injections into facet joints were first used in 1976 by Mooney and Robertson, who claimed significant long-term improvement in 52% of their patients.

The lumbar zygapophyseal joints are formed by the articulation of the inferior articular processes of one lumbar vertebra with superior articular processes of the next vertebrae. The joint exhibits the features typical of synovial joints. The articular facets are covered by articular cartilage, and a synovial membrane bridges the margins of the articular cartilage of the two facets in each joint. Surrounding the synovial membrane is a joint capsule that attaches to the articular processes a short distance beyond the margin of the articular cartilage. At the L1-4 levels, each facet joint is innervated by the medial branch of the dorsal ramus as it emerges from the intertransverse ligament and crosses the superior edge of the transverse process at its most medial end. It then passes across the root of the superior articular process. On reaching the caudal edge of the superior articular process, the medial branch hooks medially around the caudal aspect of the zygapophyseal joint. Thereafter, it courses caudal medially across the vertebral lamina. Each medial branch supplies articular branches to the caudal aspect of the joint above and to the rostral joint below. At the L5 level the dorsal ramus proper is much longer than at higher levels. The L5 dorsal ramus runs dorsally and caudally over the ala of the sacrum, lying against bone in the groove formed by the junction between the ala and the root of the superior articular processes of the sacrum.

The prevalence of chronic lumbar zygapophyseal joint pain ranges from 15% in younger patients to as high as 40% among elderly patients. The diagnosis remains one of exclusion and confirmation by analgesic injections. The clinical presentation of lumbar zygapophyseal joint–mediated pain appears to overlap considerably with the presentation of many other causes of low back pain. Most patients with lumbar zygapophyseal joint injury are neurologically intact; however, they can demonstrate pain-inhibited weakness and subjective nondermatomal extremity sensory loss and/or other sensory complaints as far distal as the foot. Patients may have exacerbation of symptoms with extension and rotation of the lumbar spine. Palpatory tenderness may be localized over the lumbar paraspinal musculature or zygapophyseal joints.

Radiographic evidence of lumbar zygapophyseal joint degeneration does not correlate with the symptoms of the disease. Bone scintigraphy has not been shown to be indicative of symptomatic zygapophyseal joint injury. CT scans, CT myelography, SPECT, and MRI scans also do not reveal whether an anatomic structure is painful or not.

The possible pathophysiology for zygapophyseal injury is **hyperextension injury**. With hyperextension, there is an increase in the load-bearing of the zygapophyseal joints, which can stretch the capsule. The mechanical deformations created from this process can also stimulate nociceptors in the facet joint capsule. Micro-trauma such as smaller articular fractures have been proposed to cause post-traumatic zygapophyseal joint pain. Lumbar zygapophyseal joint fractures, capsular tears, splits in the articular cartilage, and hemorrhage have all been documented on postmortem studies of trauma victims who had normal x-rays. Unfortunately there has been no correlation with postmortem findings to radiographs, SPECT, CT, or magnetic resonance imaging.

Clinically, patients are initially treated with anti-inflammatories, analgesics, and a graded flexion physical therapy program. There has been no research evaluating the effect of exercise therapy in proven lumbar zygapophyseal joint pain. In patients who have had persistent refractory pain and symptoms, a diagnostic **medial branch block** can be performed to access a possible cause of the patient's low back pain (see figure). Efficacy and validity of medial branch blocks have been shown. This procedure needs to be carried out under fluoroscopy with contrast to avoid venous uptake, which can occur in up to 8% of these injections. The presence of contrast also assures appropriate localization of anesthetic block of the medial branch. The exact location for the medial branch at the L1-4 levels is the dorsal surface of the transverse process just caudal to the most medial end of the superior edge of the transverse process.

Percutaneous lumbar medial branch neurotomy was initially described by Rees in 1971. He used a long scalpel blade, which was penetrated through the intertransverse ligament with the purpose of severing the posterior rami supply to the zygapophyseal joint capsule. This technique was subsequently modified by Shealy, who introduced the use of percutaneous radiofrequency electrodes in place of scalpel incisions to interrupt the nerve supply of these joints. Recently this technique has been refined to more accurately perform the neurotomy on the medial branch innervating the specific lumbar zygapophyseal joints. Several studies have now been done in a prospective randomized fashion and have shown that **radiofrequency lumbar zygapophyseal joint denervation** results in a significant reduction of pain and functional disability if it is performed in patients carefully selected on the basis of controlled diagnostic blocks.

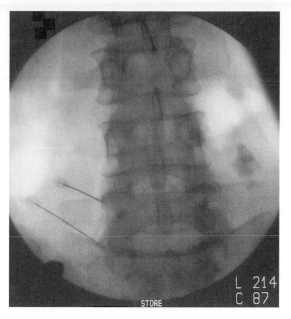

Needle placement for an L4 medial branch block and L5 dorsal ramus block.

Clinical Pearls

1. Lumbar zygapophyseal joint injury is a diagnosis of exclusion when all other causes of low back pain have been eliminated.

2. No diagnostic imaging (radiographs, MRI, CT, SPECT, and bone scintigraphy) can help in assessing whether the zygoapophyseal joint is a source of low back pain.

3. Medial branch block under fluoroscopy with contrast can minimize false negative studies.

4. All forms of conservative therapies should be tried prior to considering radiofrequency neurotomy in the treatment of chronic lumbar zygapophyseal joint pain.

5. Radiofrequency neurotomy may be an option in the treatment of patients with chronic lumbar zygapophyseal joint pain.

REFERENCES

1. Bagduk N, Long GM: Percutaneous Lumbar Medial Branch Neurotomy a Modification of Facet Denervation. Spine 5: 193–200, 1980.
2. Dreyer SJ, Dreyfuss PH: Low Back Pain and the Zygapophyseal (Facet) Joints. Arch Phy Med Rehabil 77: 290–297,1996.
3. Dreyfuss P, Halbrook B, Pauza K, et al: Efficacy and Validity of Radiofrequency Neurotomy for Chronic Lumbar Zygopophyseal Joint Pain. Spine 25: 1270–1277, 2000.
4. Dreyfuss P, Schwarzer AC, Lau P, Bagduk N: Specificity of Lumbar Medial Branch and L5 Dorsal Ramus Blocks: A Computed Tomography Study. Spine 22: 895–902, 1997.
5. Kaplan M, Dreyfus P, Halbrook B, Bagduk N: The Ability of Lumbar Medial Branch Bocks to Anesthetize the Zygapophyseal Joint A Physiologic Challenge. Spine 23: 1847–1852, 1998.
6. Shealy CN: Facet Denervation and the Management of Back and Sciatic Pain. Clin Ortho 115: 157–164, 1976.
7. Schwarzer AC, Aprill CN, Derby R, et al: Clinical Features of Patients with Pains stemming from the Lumbar Zygapophyseal Joints: Is the Lumbar Facet Syndrome A Clinical Entity? Spine 19: 1132–1137, 1994.
8. Schwarzer AC, Wang S, Bogduk N, et al: Prevalence and Clinical Features of Lumbar Zygapophyseal Joint Pain: A Study in an Australian Population with Chronic Low Back Pain. Ann R Rheum Dis 54:100–106, 1995.

PATIENT 26

A 70-year-old man with left wrist pain

A 70-year-old, right-handed man presents with a 10- to 20-month history of left wrist pain. Many years ago he suffered a fall in which he landed on his left hand, but the standard radiographs were normal at that time. He has pain mostly on the dorsoradial aspect of the wrist, and he describes it as a constant ache. There is also minimal wrist swelling and stiffness. There is no numbness, tingling, or weakness. There is no history of elbow, shoulder, or neck pain. Past history is significant for bilateral carpal tunnel release, generalized osteoarthritis, and lower extremity joint replacements.

Physical Examination: Musculoskeletal: swelling and tenderness of left wrist on dorsal aspect, mainly over radial carpal row; slight synovial thickening; restriction of movement with pain on dorsi-flexion; decreased grip strength; no muscle atrophy. Neurologic: normal.

Measurements	Left/Right
Wrist extension (degrees)	35/50 degrees
Wrist flexion	60/70 degrees
Grip strength	45/75 (Jamar pounds)

Laboratory Findings: X-ray: see figure.

Question: What is the diagnosis?

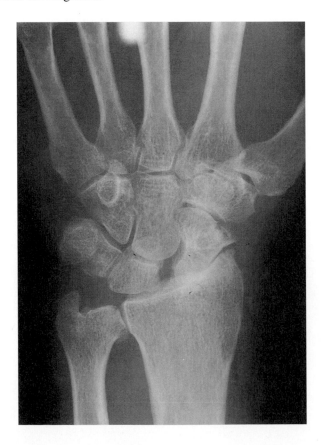

Diagnosis: Scapholunate disassociation and wrist instability

Discussion: Wrist instability is most commonly due to carpal malalignment. The carpus is considered clinically unstable if it exhibits symptomatic malalignment, is not able to bear loads, and does not have normal kinematics during any portion of its arc of motion. There is no universally acceptable classification. *Static* instability can be detected on standard wrist radiographs; however, *dynamic* instability requires stress radiographs.

In dorsal intercalated-segment instability, the proximal carpal row is *extended* with respect to the distal radius on a lateral wrist radiograph. In volar intercalated-segment instability, the proximal carpal row is *flexed* with respect to the distal radius. The proximal carpal row is defined by the long axis of the lunate.

The most common causes of wrist instability are **trauma** and **degenerative arthritis**. Scapholunate advanced collapse (SLAC) and scaphoid nonunion advanced collapse are the characteristic degeneration patterns in the wrist and represent the mechanisms by which scapholunate insufficiency and nonunion of the scaphoid occur. SLAC wrist is a gradual degeneration classified in three stages and found in post-traumatic scapholunate rupture, calcium pyrophosphate dehydrate deposition disease, rheumatoid arthritis, neuropathic diseases, trauma, and beta 2-microglobulin–associated amyloid deposition.

Scapholunate dissociation is the most frequently encountered serious ligamentous injury of the wrist. It is also a commonly missed injury. Untreated, it can lead to disabling wrist pain, reduced wrist mobility, and chronic degenerative arthritis. Early recognition of the injury by careful clinical and radiographic examination results in the most favorable prognosis. Standard posteroanterior and lateral radiographs of the wrist may be inadequate. Instead, radiographs obtained with the wrist in radial and ulnar deviation or with the hand gripping forcefully may be needed to reveal the instability of this joint.

Radionucleotide imaging, MRI, or arthrography may be required in some patients. Wrist arthroscopy is a helpful tool for the diagnosis and treatment of scapholunate instability. In fact, arthroscopy has replaced arthrography as the definitive diagnostic study for suspected carpal instability. Arthroscopy allows a detailed examination of the scapholunate interosseous and the extrinsic radiocarpal ligaments. The extent of ligamentous damage can be quantified, and a treatment algorithm can be developed based on the arthroscopic findings.

Nonoperative treatment comprises nonsteroidal anti-inflammatory medications, steroid injections, and splints. Surgical intervention is recommended for optimal results. Options include soft-tissue reconstruction, partial wrist fusion, limited carpal bone excision, or a combination of methods. Chronic injuries require specialized operative and rehabilitative management.

In the present patient, an unrecognized ligamentous injury to his left wrist was likely at the time of his fall. The onset of his symptoms was gradual, to the point where he was experiencing significant disability. X-ray revealed scapholunate dissociation and degenerative changes, most marked in the radiocarpal joint. He was treated with cortisone injections and a wrist splint. Due to the collapse and degenerative carpal disease, a limited wrist fusion was performed with only partial relief of his symptoms.

Clinical Pearls

1. Wrist instability is unrecognized in at least 5% of soft tissue wrist injuries.

2. The most common mechanism of injury is falling on an outstretched hand, leading to acute ligament injuries, fractures, and dislocations

3. Seven initial radiographs are recommended for diagnosis, including posteroanterior, lateral, radial and ulnar deviation, flexion and extension, and a clenched fist view.

4. Arthroscopic evaluation of the wrist is more accurate and specific than arthrography for diagnosis of wrist ligament injury.

5. Optimal management is surgical, depending on the patient's symptoms and the extent of ligament damage and instability.

REFERENCES

1. Atkinson LS, Baxley EG: Scapholunate dissociation. Am Fam Physician 49:1845–1850, 1994.
2. Gelberman RH, Cooney WP, Szabo RM: Carpal instability. Instructional course lecture. J Bone Joint Surg 82A:578–594, 2000.
3. The Anatomy and Biomechanics Committee of the International Federation of Societies for the Surgery of the Hand: Definition of carpal instability. J. Hand Surg 24A:866–867, 1999.
4. Wintman BI, Gelberman RH, Katz JN: Dynamic scapholunate instability: results of operative treatment with dorsal capsulodesis. J Hand Surg 20A:971–979, 1995.

PATIENT 27

A 71-year-old man with chronic knee pain

A 71-year-old man who has been experiencing left knee pain for 10 years presents with progressive pain and inability to walk long distances. Over the last year, the patient has had to reduce his walking program from two miles to approximately one-quarter of a mile. Recently, he began using a single-point cane in his right hand, which has provided minimal relief. He denies locking or catching of the joint, but does experience intermittent swelling. He has been unable to tolerate nonsteroidal anti-inflammatory drugs (NSAIDs) due to gastritis, and instead uses acetaminophen (1000 mg PO qid) for pain control. The patient reports some history of shoulder and hip pain, but no limitation of activities that require arm use. Past medical history includes mild hypertension, gastroesophageal reflux disease, and gastritis.

Physical Examination: General: well-developed, appears stated age. Cardiac: regular rate and rhythm, without murmur. Chest: clear to auscultation. Abdomen: benign. Musculoskeletal: posture reveals mild thoracic kyphosis; strength of upper extremities 5/5 throughout; strength of lower extremities 4+/5 left quadriceps, otherwise 5/5 throughout; on active range of motion (ROM), left knee flexion limited to 110 degrees and extension to –10 degrees; painful arc of motion and crepitus on passive ROM; mild bony hypertrophy of knee; anterior and posterior drawer signs negative; McMurray's sign negative. Skin: no effusion.

Laboratory Findings: Rheumatoid factor negative. ANA negative. ESR negative, CBC and electrolytes normal. Radiographs (*see figure*): changes of osteoarthritis in left knee, including loss of medial joint space and osteophytes on medial tibial plateau; subchondral cyst on tibial surface.

Question: Other than pharmacotherapy, what are nonsurgical treatment alternatives for this patient's osteoarthritis of the knee?

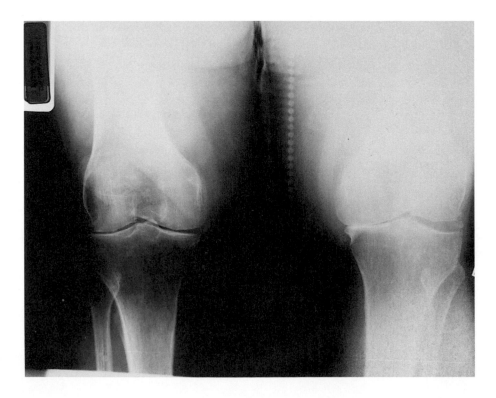

Answer: Exercise and viscosupplementation with hyaluronic acid

Discussion: Osteoarthritis is one of the most common diseases affecting the U.S. population today. Approximately 16 million Americans suffer from this disorder. Eighty percent of people older than 55 years of age have radiographic evidence of osteoarthritis. It is estimated that there are 73 million doctor visits and 36 million days lost from work each year due to osteoarthritis and its complications.

Known factors associated with the development of osteoarthritis include **trauma to a joint** and **repetitive stress** activities. Osteoarthritis of the knee has also been found to have an association with weakness of the quadriceps muscle group. A correlation exists between joints used in activities and the development of osteoarthritis. Obesity has also been reported to be a contributing factor in the development of bilateral osteoarthritis of the knee. One study reported that with weight loss of five kilograms, a 50% reduction of symptoms of osteoarthritis was seen.

The signs and symptoms associated with osteoarthritis include morning stiffness that improves with activity and a gel phenomenon that occurs with periods of inactivity, leading to transient stiffness. The diagnosis of osteoarthritis of the knee is usually supported by characteristic findings on plain radiographs. These changes, as in the present patient, include loss of joint space, osteophytes, subchondral bony sclerosis, and subchondral cysts. Local signs of inflammation such as redness, warmth, and effusion are sometimes present, but are much less prevalent than in the inflammatory arthropathies. Specific examination of the joints involved is also important. Limited range of motion, crepitus, and valgus/varus deformities of the knees are sometimes present.

Exercise is an integral part of the treatment of osteoarthritis. Aerobic exercise not only improves cardiovascular fitness, but has been shown to reduce pain and improve functional mobility in patients with osteoarthritis. Studies have also shown that strengthening of the quadriceps can decrease pain and increase function in osteoarthritis of the knee. In addition to acetaminophen, the first-line pharmacologic therapy, the AMA guides and the American College of Rheumatology emphasize the role of rehabilitation therapies in the management of osteoarthritis. A comprehensive program including the guidance of physical and occupational therapists should be implemented. Emphasis should be on strength training, improved range of motion, and the use of appropriate assistive devices and joint protective techniques. Thermal modalities including hot packs and ice massage can be used as an adjunct to therapy to improve relaxation.

In addition to acetaminophen, NSAIDs have been used extensively to treat osteoarthritis. However, in older patients the side effects of these medications (e.g., GI bleed, renal dysfunction, and mental status changes) often prohibit long-term use. With the development of the new COX2 receptor inhibitors, perhaps a safer alternative has been established.

For patients who have failed conservative therapy, but are not eligible for surgery, **viscosupplementation** with hyaluronic acid is a viable alternative. Viscosupplementation is also used to delay surgery for an extended period of time. This procedure, approved in 1997 by the FDA, involves the intra-articular injection of a synthetically produced hyaluronic acid. Two commercial preparations are available in the U.S. The injection of hyaluronic acid into the knees of patients with osteoarthritis decreases pain—possibly because of an effect on the intra-articular pain receptors. One of the more simple postulations is that the injections improve the lubrication of the intra-articular surfaces as well as enhance the elasticity and viscosity of the synovial fluid. Viscosupplementation with hyaluronic acid also inhibits inflammatory mediators that are thought to play a role in the pathophysiology of osteoarthritis.

The injections are usually given in a series of three to five weekly rounds. If a favorable outcome is achieved, repeat treatment is considered usually after 6 months to 1 year. Viscosupplementation is contraindicated for patients in whom a septic joint cannot be ruled out. Side effects are infrequent but can include local irritation or infection, headache, or GI complaints. There is no evidence to conclude that hyaluronic acid arrests the progression of the disease; however, its pain-reducing properties have been proven.

Clinical Pearls

1. Comprehensive management of osteoarthritis (OA) should include physical and occupational therapies.

2. Goals of OA management are maximizing functional movement of joints, pain relief, and appropriate use of assistive devices.

3. Viscosupplementation using hyaluronic acid appears to be a safe and effective alternative for treatment of osteoarthritis.

4. Injection of hyaluronic acid into the knee decreases pain secondary to osteoarthritis, possibly by its effect on intra-articular pain receptors and inhibition of inflammatory mediators.

REFERENCES

1. Cefalu CA, Waddell DS: Viscosupplementation: Treatment alternative for osteoarthritis of the knee. Geriatrics 54(10):51–57, 1999.
2. Rehman Q, Lane NE: Getting control of osteoarthritis pain. An update on treatment options. Postgrad Med 106(4):127–134, 1999.
3. Schwartz ST, Zimmermann B: Update of Osteoarthritis. Med Health R I 82(9):321-324, 1999.

PATIENT 28

A 52-year-old woman with arm swelling post mastectomy

A 52-year-old woman initially presented to her general practitioner because she noticed asymmetry to her breasts; an unusual, bumpy texture to the right breast; and partial inversion of the right nipple. She told her doctor that she had not noticed any recent fever, chills, night sweats, or weight loss. She did report having been unusually tired during the past 2 months.

Physical Examination: Vital signs: normal. Abdomen: soft, nontender, normal bowel sounds. Cardiac: regular rate, no murmurs. Extremities: no swelling, cyanosis, or numbness. Motor: intact, except for trace weakness in proximal lower extremity and upper extremity muscles. Breasts: right breast slightly elevated relative to left; partially retracted right nipple, but no discharge; orange peel texture of skin; hard, nontender, and relatively immobile lump approximately 5 cm in diameter just posterior to nipple; two right axillary nodes swollen and tender.

Laboratory Findings: Mammogram: one spherical mass, 7 cm in diameter, posterior to right nipple; left breast normal. Biopsy of mass: malignant cells. *Referral to oncology surgeon*—Biopsy of swollen axillary lymph node: malignant cells. CT scan of chest, abdomen, brain, and axillary regions: tumor in center of right breast; suspicious-looking axillary lymph nodes on right.

Course: The patient was counseled at great length by the surgeon regarding her various options, and she opted for the mastectomy with axillary node dissection. She received postoperative radiation therapy. Within 2 weeks of surgery, painful swelling occurred in the entire right upper extremity. The swelling transiently resolved for 3 weeks, but then recurred.

Question: What is the cause of the arm swelling?

Diagnosis: Lymphedema resulting from the axillary lymph node/lymphatic tissue resections

Discussion: Incidence of all the major forms of cancer, with the exception of stomach and cervical tumors, has been increasing during the past 40 years. Breast cancer remains the leading cause of mortality in women 40–55 years old, and it accounts for 18% of all cancer deaths in women. Lymphedema occurs in over 38% of patients who have undergone mastectomy with axillary node clearance. Patients who receive radiation therapy postoperatively are believed to have a higher incidence of lymphedema than do patients who do not receive radiation treatment. Other complications following this surgery include chest wall pain, pectoral weakness (especially if the pectorals are removed during the surgery), reduced shoulder range of motion, cellulitis and infection to the edematous arm, and, several months to years following radiation treatment, brachial plexopathy.

Treatment of lymphedema comprises two major categories: nonoperative and operative. With the exception of refractory cases, nonoperative treatments are preferred over surgical procedures. These conservative measures include physical therapy, diuretics, diet alterations, antimicrobials, and, to a lesser extent, immunologic therapy and mesotherapy (injection of a hyaluronidase-type agent to loosen the extracellular matrix). The most widely accepted treatment is **multimodal physical therapy.** The emphasis here is on treatment and prevention. The lymphedema is reduced by the use of massage, compression bandaging and garments, and pneumatic compression pumps. Range of motion and strengthening are also incorporated into the therapy program. (See references for more detailed discussions of other conservative treatments and surgical options.)

Psychological support is of great importance for people living with any form of cancer. It is estimated that up to 50% of people with cancer meet the criteria for clinical depression. The patient's body image changes due to the mastectomy, and lymphedema can negatively impact overall confidence. Psychological counseling should be offered to these patients. Cosmetic options include breast prostheses and reconstructive surgery; these should be discussed with the patient.

The present patient's lymphedema was addressed with a combination of garment and manual compression, along with pneumatic compression, and the majority of the lymphedema resolved within 2 weeks. However, she was aware that the therapeutic interventions she implemented would need to be continued indefinitely. She then opted for a prosthesis. Her cancer has been in remission for 5 years. Brachial plexopathy did occur to the upper trunk of her brachial plexus 1 year post radiation. Physical therapy has restored moderate strength to her biceps and periscapular muscles. She wears a compression garment on her right arm and uses a pneumatic compression pump every other day. Her husband helps her with retrograde massage on the other days.

Clinical Pearls

1. Breast cancer is the leading cause of mortality in women 40–55 years old.

2. Lymphedema occurs in at least 38% of patients following mastectomy with axillary clearance, and the incidence increases in those who receive radiation treatment postoperatively.

3. Radiation brachial plexopathy may be delayed for over 20 years.

4. Nonoperative treatments incorporating massage, pneumatic pumps, and compression garments have been the mainstay of treatment for post-mastectomy lymphedema.

5. Approximately 50% of patients with cancer meet the criteria for clinical depression.

REFERENCES
1. Brennan MJ, DePompolo RW, Garden FH: Focused review: Postmastectomy lymphedema. Arch Phys Med Rehabil 77: S74–S79, 1996.
2. Cole RP, Scialla SJ, Bednarz L: Functional recovery in cancer rehabilitation. Arch Phys Med Rehabil 81:623–627, 2000.
3. Garden FH, Gillis TA: Principles of cancer rehabilitation. In Braddom RL (ed): Physical Medicine and Rehabilitation. Philadelphia, WB Saunders Company, 1996, pp 1199–1214.

PATIENT 29

A 4-year-old boy with abnormal posture

A 4-year-old boy was noted by his parents to have "an unusual way of standing." No other specific problems were presented to the patient's pediatrician on a routine physical exam. Following routine evaluation, and on the insistence of the patient's parents, the child was referred for physiatric evaluation of an abnormal posture. Specifically, the parents wanted to know if there were any exercises that could be prescribed to improve the boy's posture.

Physical Examination: General: well-nourished, well-developed; no acute distress. Chest: normal. Abdomen: round, soft, nontender.

Musculoskeletal: only moderate increased lumbar lordosis; slightly enlarged calf muscles.

Laboratory Findings: CPK: normal to just under 7000 IU/L. Muscle biopsy (see figure): necrosis and differing muscle fiber size. Immunohistochemistry: mild/partial dystrophin deficiency, determined by positive (normal) staining in all fibers with dys2 and dys3 but poor staining with dys1 (rod domain) in majority of fibers. DNA analysis: deletion at exons 45–47.

Questions: What is the diagnosis? What kind of exercises should be prescribed or avoided?

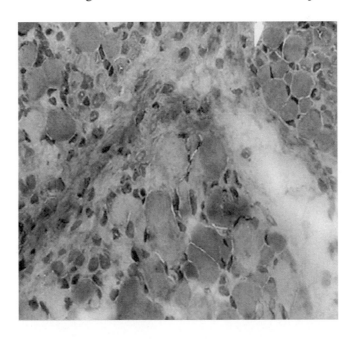

Answers: Becker's muscular dystrophy. Avoid eccentric exercises.

Discussion: While the history and physical exam were rather unrevealing, the lab tests indicated a diagnosis of Becker's muscular dystrophy. A deletion at exons 45–47 of the dystrophin gene is one of the more common deletions resulting in the milder Becker's muscular dystrophy phenotype, rather than the lethal Duchenne's muscular dystrophy phenotype. Becker's is variable in clinical outcome, but most often mild, and most patients still walk well into middle age or beyond. In contrast, Duchenne's muscular dystrophy (DMD) is a devastating, inherited muscle disease affecting 1/3500 live male births worldwide. Affected boys become progressively weak due to muscle wasting and contractures, frequently leading to wheelchair use by the age of 12. Dystrophin, the deficient protein in DMD, is normally located on the internal surface of the myofiber membrane.

The mild lumbar lordosis and calf hypertrophy noted in the present patient resulted from differential expression of disease among muscles, likely due to a number of factors including posture and muscle use. Importantly, some forms of muscular contraction probably induce muscle damage to a greater degree in dystrophic muscle compared to normal. Investigators have noted that dystrophin deficiency leads to differential pathological involvement of affected muscle. Indeed, selective involvement of the iliotibial tract has been proposed to cause premature loss of ambulation in DMD patients. In dystrophic (*mdx*) mice, muscles demonstrated (**1**) greater penetration of membrane-impermeable dye immediately after lengthening (eccentric) contractions, and (**2**) an increased rate of necrosis than was seen in controls immediately following lengthening contractions.

While the role of exercise in muscular dystrophies is not yet clear, the evidence described above suggests that eccentric exercises should generally be avoided in patients with Becker's or Duchenne's muscular dystrophy. Therefore, an exercise prescription should include precautions regarding eccentric contractions in these patients.

Clinical Pearls

1. Some muscles are preferentially injured in Duchenne's muscular dystrophy (DMD). Reasons for this selective muscle involvement are complex, but likely involve muscular use and posture.

2. Eccentric (lengthening) exercises are likely to lead to greater than normal injury in DMD patients.

REFERENCES

1. Cullen MJ, Walsh J, Nicholson LV, Harris JB: Ultrastructural localization of dystrophin in human muscle by using gold immunolabeling. Proceedings of the Royal Society of London - Series B: Biological Sciences 240:197–210, 1990.
2. Johnson EW: The iliotibial band—a malignant structure masquerading as benign [editorial]. Am J Phys Med Rehabil 76:1–1, 1997.
3. Kornegay JN, Sharp NJ, Schueler RO, Betts CW: Tarsal joint contracture in dogs with golden retriever muscular dystrophy. Lab Anim Sci 44:331–333, 1994.
4. Monaco AP: Molecular human genetics and the Duchenne/Becker muscular dystrophy gene. In Partridge T (ed): Molecular and Cell Biology of Muscular Dystrophy. London, Chapman & Hall,1993, pp 1–8.
5. Petrof BJ, Shrager JB, Stedman HH, et al: Dystrophin protects the sarcolemma from stresses developed during muscle contraction. Proc Natl Acad Sci 90:3710–3714, 1993.
6. Valentine BA, Cooper BJ: Canine X-linked muscular dystrophy: Selective involvement of muscles in neonatal dogs. Neuromuscular Disorders 1:31–38, 1991.
7. Watkins SC, Hoffman EP, Slayter HS, Kunkel LM: Immunoelectron microscopic localization of dystrophin in myofibres. Nature 333:863–866, 1988.
8. Weller B, Karpati G, Carpenter S: Dystrophin-deficient mdx muscle fibers are preferentially vulnerable to necrosis induced by experimental lengthening contractions. J Neurol Sci 100:9–13, 1990.

PATIENT 30

A 75-year-old man with wrist pain and swelling

A 75-year-old man presents with left wrist pain and swelling, which he has been experiencing for several years. He denies any history of numbness, paresthesia, or weakness of his hand or upper limbs. There is no history of recent trauma, but he reports sustaining a fracture of the left wrist joint many years ago. He has noticed no swelling or pain of other joints. His past medical history is significant for hypertension, adult-onset diabetes mellitus, hypothyroidism, benign prostatic hyperplasia, and depression.

Physical Examination: Extremities: no joint deformity or swelling; Tinel's sign not elicited at either wrist joint. Musculoskeletal: weakness of left abductor pollicis brevis (3/5); normal strength in all other muscles (5/5). Neurologic: hypesthesia to light touch in left index and middle fingers; Achilles reflexes absent; all other deep tendon reflexes present and symmetric bilaterally.

Laboratory Findings: See results of nerve conduction and EMG studies below.

Question: What is the diagnosis?

Nerve Conduction Study

Nerves	Site	Latency	Amplitude	CV
Sensory				
Left median	Wrist	4.4 msec	24 µV	31.8 m/s
Left ulnar	Wrist	NR	—	—
Left median (Bactrian)	Wrist	3.3 msec	15 µV	30.3 m/s
Left radial (Bactrian)	Wrist	2.3 msec	8 µV	43.5 m/s
Right median (Bactrian)	Wrist	2.9 msec	13 µV	34.5 m/s
Right radial (Bactrian)	Wrist	2.4 msec	7 µV	41.7 m/s
Left sural	Ankle	NR	—	—
Right sural	Ankle	NR	—	—
Motor				
Left median	Wrist	4.8 msec	7.1 mV	—
	Elbow	—	5.9 mV	57.1 m/s
Right median	Wrist	4.3 msec	8.1 mV	—
	Elbow	—	8.0 mV	56.0 m/s
Left ulnar	Wrist	3.6 msec	8.6 mV	—
	Below elbow	—	7.3 mV	52.3 m/s
	Above elbow	—	6.9 mV	51.4 m/s
Right peroneal	Ankle	4.8 msec	2.0 mV	—
	Fib head	—	1.9 mV	35.6 m/s

NR = no response; Normal Med – Rad difference is < 0.6 ms; Bactrian = test that compares radial and median sensory nerves

EMG Study

Muscle	Ins Act	Fibs	PSW	Fasc.	MUAP Morph	IP
Left APB	Normal	1+	1+	None	Normal	Full
Left FDI	Normal	None	None	None	Normal	Full
Left PT	Normal	None	None	None	Normal	Full
Right APB	Normal	None	None	None	Normal	Full

Ins Act = insertional activity, Fibs = fibrillation potentials, PSW = positive sharp waves, Fasc = fasciculations, MUAP Morph = motor unit action potential morphology, IP = interference pattern, APB = abductor pollicis brevis, FDI = first dorsal interosseous, PT = pronator teres

Diagnosis: Left carpal tunnel syndrome with demyelinating sensory polyneuropathy

Discussion: Carpal tunnel syndrome (CTS) is a symptom complex that includes numbness and paresthesias in the hand and stinging, burning, or aching pain that may extend proximally to the elbow or even up to the shoulder. Symptoms typically worsen at night, often to the point of waking the patient. Symptoms may worsen with manual activities such as knitting, using hand tools, or driving a car. In advanced cases, the first four digits may have severely impaired sensation, and the thenar eminence may be atrophied. The differential diagnosis of these symptoms includes cervical radiculopathy, polyneuropathy, brachial plexopathy, ulnar mononeuropathy, proximal median neuropathy, amyotrophic lateral sclerosis, and central nervous system lesions such as cerebral infarction and multiple sclerosis.

An electrodiagnostic exam is frequently requested to confirm the diagnosis of CTS. A variety of sensitive motor and sensory nerve conduction studies (NCS) can be used to evaluate suspected CTS. Motor NCS of the median nerve show a prolonged distal latency in 60–74 % of patients who are clinically suspected to have CTS. In approximately 10% of patients, median motor nerve conduction velocity is slowed in the forearm, usually in association with prolongation of the distal motor latency. Comparison of the median motor distal latency (recording from the second lumbrical muscle) with the ulnar motor distal latency (recording from the dorsal interosseus muscle) increases the sensitivity of the study.

Median sensory NCS may be performed orthodromically or antidromically. With the conduction study performed between the wrist and a digit, 49–66% of patients with CTS demonstrate either a prolonged median sensory peak distal latency or absent median sensory nerve action potential. With short segment incremental (inching) median sensory NCS across the carpal tunnel, 81% of patients also demonstrate abnormalities. Comparison studies of median and ulnar sensory conduction and median and radial sensory conduction improve diagnostic sensitivity. Of patients with CTS, 82% demonstrate abnormalities with median and ulnar sensory conduction between wrist and ring finger, and 60–69% demonstrate abnormalities in comparison of median and radial sensory conduction between wrist and thumb. Median mixed NCS performed between the wrist and palm are abnormal in 69–84% of patients with CTS.

Needle examination helps to define the severity of the lesion by indicating the presence of axonal destruction as manifested by abnormal spontaneous activity. Prolonged median motor and sensory distal latencies are the most important predictors of an abnormal needle examination of the abductor pollicis brevis.

Individuals with polyneuropathy are susceptible to focal trauma. Therefore, it is not unusual to find a clinical mononeuropathy *superimposed* upon a mild polyneuropathy. Up to one-third of patients with diabetes mellitus have electrodiagnostic evidence of a median mononeuropathy. Electrodiagnosis of polyneuropathy requires both motor and sensory conduction studies, preferably in at least three limbs. Bilateral studies should be performed on several peripheral nerves to demonstrate the characteristic symmetry of abnormality. In those patients with mild to moderate symptoms and signs, conduction studies should be performed on the most involved site and, in those with severe signs and symptoms, on the least involved site.

Needle electromyography is useful in grossly defining the chronicity of an axonal lesion. It is also useful in identifying other disorders that may be superimposed or confused with polyneuropathy. Recommendation for the needle examination in a suspected polyneuropathy includes examination of the anterior tibialis, medial gastrocnemius, first dorsal interosseous, and lumbar paraspinal muscles. Any abnormality should be confirmed by examination of one contralateral muscle. If examination is normal, the intrinsic foot muscles should be examined.

There are no clear guidelines on electrodiagnostic evaluation in cases of mononeuropathies in those patients with superimposed peripheral neuropathy. When a peripheral neuropathy is confirmed electrodiagnostically, CTS can still be diagnosed if the median motor and sensory distal latencies are disproportionately prolonged compared with the ulnar or radial distal latencies. Segmental nerve conduction techniques that demonstrate slowing of conduction in the transcarpal segment, but not in the palm-to-digit or forearm segments, may be helpful, but need to be interpreted with caution.

In the present patient, clinical history and exam encouraged suspicion of median neuropathy and peripheral neuropathy. The NCS revealed prolonged left median nerve distal latency and absent sensory action potentials in the lower extremities. Needle electromyography revealed evidence of axonal destruction of the median nerve affecting the abductor pollicis brevis. Both of these findings confirmed the diagnosis.

Clinical Pearls

1. Carpal tunnel syndrome (CTS) is a commonly encountered entity and one of the most frequent reasons for referral to an electrodiagnostic laboratory.

2. In the presence of a polyneuropathy, patients are susceptible to focal mononeuropathies.

3. A variety of nerve conduction studies are available for evaluation of patients when there is clinical suspicion of CTS. The individual choice of tests depends on the experience of the electromyographer and is dictated by any superimposed conditions and clinical examination.

4. There are no clear guidelines for evaluation of CTS in patients with peripheral neuropathy. Up to one-third of patients with diabetes mellitus have electrodiagnostic evidence of distal median nerve compression.

REFERENCES

1. AAEM Quality Assurance Committee: Literature review of the usefulness of nerve conduction studies and electromyography for the evaluation of patients with carpal tunnel syndrome. Muscle Nerve 16:1392–1414, 1993.
2. Donofrio PD, Albers JW: AAEM minimonograph # 34: Polyneuropathy: Classification by nerve conduction studies and electromyography. Muscle Nerve 13:889–903, 1990.
3. Hawley RJ: Frequency of median mononeuropathy in patients with mild diabetic neuropathy in the early diabetes intervention trial. Muscle Nerve 19:1504–1505, 1996.
4. Stevens JC.: AAEM minimonograph # 26: The electrodiagnosis of carpal tunnel syndrome. Muscle Nerve 20:1477–1486, 1997.
5. Vogt T, Mika A, Thomke F, Hopf HC: Evaluation of carpal tunnel syndrome in patients with polyneuropathy. Muscle Nerve 20:153–157, 1997.

PATIENT 31

A 53-year-old woman with left hemiplegia, left upper extremity pain, and swelling

A 53-year-old, hypertensive woman recently suffered a hemorrhagic stroke. She sustained left hemiplegia, with a muscle grade of 0/5 in the left upper and lower extremities. Left hemi-neglect was also noted. Two weeks later, while undergoing rehabilitation, progressive swelling and burning pain in the left forearm and hand occurred over a period of about 3 days. The patient thinks that she may have accidentally hit her left side while performing bathroom transfers prior to the appearance of these symptoms. She complains of constant pain in the entire extremity, especially in the shoulder, both at rest and with range of motion.

Physical Examination: Blood pressure 155/90, pulse 80, respirations 17, temperature 99.2°. General: alert; mild distress due to left upper extremity pain. Skin: mild swelling, redness, and coolness of left hand compared to right. Neurologic: light touch elicited complaints of pain. Musculoskeletal: +1 pitting edema; marked tenderness, especially at the metacarpal joint; no palpable or visible movement in left upper extremity, as well as evidence of neglect. Attempts at range of motion elicited requests from patient not to continue with this part of exam.

Laboratory Findings: WBC 10,800/µl, hemoglobin 11.3 g/dl, Hct 33%, platelet count 226,000/µl. ESR 58 mm/hr. X-rays of left shoulder: negative for fracture or dislocation. X-rays of left wrist and hand: soft tissue swelling; no fracture or dislocation. Venous Doppler: negative for venous thrombosis. Bone scan: asymmetric uptake in blood flow and blood pool phases; increased periarticular uptake in delayed images.

Question: What is the cause of the patient's upper extremity pain and swelling?

Diagnosis: Complex regional pain syndrome type I

Discussion: A patient with hemiplegia from any number of causes (e.g., thrombotic stroke, intracerebral hemorrhage, traumatic brain injury, brain tumor) can develop swelling of an extremity. This event requires an investigation on the part of the treating physician. The most important differential diagnoses include fracture, venous thrombosis, and reflex sympathetic dystrophy (RSD), now preferably termed complex regional pain syndrome (CRPS) type I.

In this patient, a history of trauma was elicited; hence, a possible fracture needs to be ruled out. It is important to remember that x-rays may be negative during the first week after the inciting event.

Venous thrombosis, especially in the deep venous system, is another serious entity that should be considered. A venous Doppler study is useful and non-invasive. It has 96% sensitivity and 98% specificity in symptomatic patients. Venography remains the gold standard, but it is invasive, expensive, and has the potential for untoward reactions; therefore, it used only when clinically warranted.

CRPS type I has been reported in 12–25% of hemiplegic stroke patients, and is the only common cause of shoulder pain at rest. Several diagnostic criteria have been published for RSD. Most describe distal swelling and pain out of proportion to injury. The syndrome also includes hyperalgesia, trophic changes, and vasomotor instability. Three stages have been described:

Acute (3-6 months)—deep, burning pain, worse with movement; soft edema; redness; initial hyperthermia; and, later, hypothermia and hyperhidrosis. Bone demineralization begins at this stage, but x-rays are usually normal. The 3-phase bone scan may be positive, with 60% sensitivity and 80% specificity. If positive, it will show asymmetric uptake in the blood flow and blood pool phases and increased periarticular uptake in the delayed images, as in the present patient. Up to 40% of patients with CRPS type I have negative bone scans.

Atrophic (6-9 months)—increased pain intensity, spreading proximally; brawny edema with mottling of the skin and brittle nails; decreased range of motion; and early atrophy. Patchy periarticular osteopenia may be seen on x-ray, but this occurs in only about 50% of patients. The bone scan may still be positive.

Dystrophic (> 9 months to years)—pain may continue, increase, or subside except with movement. The involved hand or foot is pale, cool, and dry, with a smooth, shiny appearance. Muscle atrophy and joint contractures are present. X-rays show diffuse osteoporosis.

The gold standard for diagnosis of CRPS type I is relief of pain with a stellate ganglion block.

Treatment regimens can become complex, and include medications (such as NSAIDs, steroid dosepaks, beta-blockers, tricyclic antidepressants), intra-articular injections, topicals, physical therapy (also physical modalities), as well as the already mentioned stellate ganglion block. Frequently, the condition becomes prolonged enough to warrant comprehensive chronic pain management.

Clinical Pearls

1. Complex regional pain syndrome (CRPS) type I is the only common cause of shoulder pain at rest in hemiplegic stroke patients.
2. The bone scan is only 60% sensitive and 80% specific in diagnosing CRPS type I.
3. The gold standard for diagnosis of CRPS type I is a stellate ganglion block.

REFERENCES
1. Black-Schaffer RM, Kirsteins AE, Harvey RL: Stroke rehabilitation. 2. Comorbidities and complications. Arch Phys Med Rehabil 80:S8–S16, 1999.
2. Fournier RS, Holder LE: Reflex sympathetic dystrophy: Diagnostic controversies. Semin Nucl Med 28(1):116–123, 1998.
3. Murray IPC, Ell PJ (eds): Nuclear Medicine in Clinical Diagnosis and Treatment, 2nd ed. Edinburgh, Churchill-Livingstone, 1998.
4. Slaten W, O'Connor K: Reflex sympathetic dystrophy. In O'Young B, Young MA, Stiens SA (eds): PM&R Secrets. Philadelphia, Hanley and Belfus, 1997, pp 360-364.

PATIENT 32

A teenager with hip pain and malposition after anoxic encephalopathy

A 13-year-old girl presents to follow-up approximately 1 year after a severe anoxic event. The anoxia was caused by an asthma exacerbation, for which she was transported to the hospital by private vehicle. She suffered a 10- to 12-minute respiratory arrest in the process. Her initial head CT scan in the pediatric ICU showed global cerebral edema and herniation; a repeat showed occipital hypodensity and some resolution of the edema. She survived and was discharged to home in a minimally responsive condition with limited equipment and nursing care; home health therapists felt they had no goals and discontinued services.

At this visit, the patient's family is concerned about scoliosis and lower extremity contractures. Over the last few months, she has experienced increasing discomfort with sitting, and her nurse believes that there has been some asymmetry in posture since about 6–7 months post injury. There is no history of prior or subsequent trauma. The patient is taking baclofen 10 mg TID and Zanaflex 4 mg TID as antispasticity medication and also uses resting splints for foot and ankle positioning in her wheelchair. She sits in her wheelchair with significant pelvic rotation and obliquity despite a Jay positioning cushion with abductor and hip guides; her right side is high and forward, which tends to obscure right hip contracture and shorter leg somewhat. Her asthma has been stable on Flovent and albuterol. She has a tracheostomy and is tube fed, as a videofluoroscopic swallowing study showed that conditions were unfavorable for resuming oral feeding despite clinical return of the swallowing reflex. Of note, she has just experienced menarche. Her hygiene and overall care is clearly excellent.

Physical Examination: General: responsive to verbal and tactile input with facial expression, eye opening, and minimal movements of her left arm at times. Spine: long, partly flexible C-curve. Abdomen: normal; gastrostomy tube in good condition. Musculoskeletal: upper extremity flexion contractures at both wrists and elbows; hamstrings allow 100–105° popliteal angles; mild equinovalgus contracture of both feet and ankles; significant adduction contracture of right hip, 20° short of neutral, and right femur shorter.

Laboratory Findings: Radiograph of hips: see figure below.

Question: What is the diagnosis?

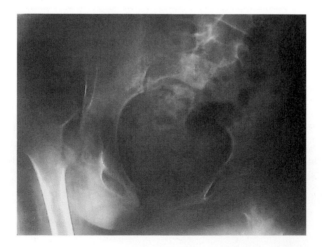

Diagnosis: Hip dislocation.

Discussion: This is a strikingly unusual event for a child of this age. Our pediatric PM&R service saw a similar event in a 10-year-old boy about 18 months post severe brain and brainstem injury, with return of responsiveness but very limited motor control, with severe spastic quadriplegia (see figure below.) His dislocation occurred over the course of about 3 months and was similarly painful, requiring surgical intervention. Note that his hip stayed in place for over a year with regular physical therapy, but therapy had ceased just prior to this 3-month period.

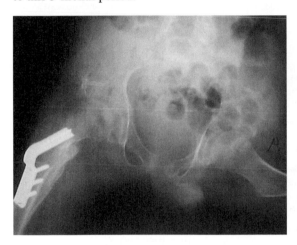

The present patient also required surgical intervention; a Schantz osteotomy and adductor and flexor tendon releases were performed initially, followed by additional releases about 6 months later, including left hip flexor release with anterior capsulotomy, left medial hamstring lengthening, and bilateral percutaneous heel cord lengthening. An intrathecal baclofen trial undertaken as a potential aid in preventing repeat dislocation was not effective in reducing tone. Home health services were informed that non-provision of therapy services could contribute to recurrence. Physical therapy was reinstated.

An additional example of this type of injury is seen below, in a 4-year-old girl with traumatic brain and brainstem injury. She had extremely severe tone, and her hip dislocated out of a previously normal acetabulum several months after injury.

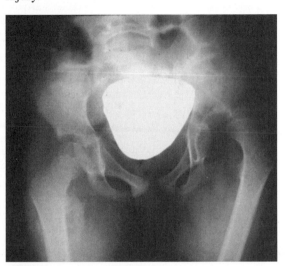

Clinical Pearls

1. Children's hips are at risk proportional to severity of adductor and flexor tone—less so as they approach the age of bony maturity, but still vulnerable.

2. A previously normal hip (i.e., one without acetabular dysplasia or coxa valga) requires more extraordinary forces to cause dislocation than one that has developed abnormally under the influence of abnormal muscular forces.

3. Families tend to report discomfort rather than asymmetry of trunk and hip or pelvic position; family and staff tend to position the patient based on femur length (knee position) looking symmetrical. Custom-molded rather than modular seating may provide better control, as well as visual cues to indicate accommodation of any leg length difference.

4. Therapy may reduce tone and abnormal forces, thereby preventing or delaying progression of subluxation.

REFERENCES
1. Abrams RA, Mubarak S: Musculoskeletal consequences of near-drowning in children. J Pediatr Orthop 11(2):168–175, 1991.
2. Blasier D, Letts RM: Pediatric update #7. The orthopaedic manifestations of head injury in children. Orthop Rev 18(3):350–358, 1989.

PATIENT 33

A 38-year-old man with fever and tetraplegia

A 38-year-old man experienced a flu-like illness and generalized body aches and fatigue approximately 1 month ago, and he was started on Augmentin. One day later, an erythematous rash on his left forearm and fever developed, so his local physician gave him an intramuscular injection of Rocephin, and he was discharged to home. However, his fever continued and he developed right shoulder weakness and pain, which progressed to left shoulder weakness and eventually bilateral lower extremity weakness over the next week. When he fell and was unable to get up his family called an ambulance, and he was then admitted to the local hospital for work-up. Over the next several days urinary retention and constipation developed. When he started to develop shortness of breath, he was transferred to the university hospital.

Physical Examination: Temperature 102.2°; pulse 96; respirations 32; blood pressure 144/68. HEENT: neck stiff and resistant to any movement in all directions. Chest: normal. Cardiac: normal. Abdomen: nontender, with normal active bowel sounds. Musculoskeletal: full range of motion of upper and lower extremities. Skin: 13×15 cm, warm, erythematous, and blanchable rash on left arm. Neurologic: flaccid muscle tone and absent muscle stretch reflexes of upper and lower extremities; 0/5 strength in bilateral upper and lower extremities, except for trace shoulder abduction strength bilaterally; absent sensation to pinprick and light touch distal to C5 dermatome on right and C3 dermatome on left. Rectal: weak voluntary anal sphincter contraction; deep pressure sensation present, but no sensation to pinprick or light touch.

Laboratory Findings: WBC 21,000/μl with 84% neutrophils (75% segs and 7% bands); hct 39.3 %; platelets 363,000/ml. Sodium 125, creatinine 1.7 mg/dl, CPK 691 mg/dl. Urinalysis: normal except for 1+ blood. Lyme antibody: positive. Blood cultures: methicillin-resistant *Staphylococcus aureus*. Chest x-ray: no active pulmonary disease. CT scan of head: normal. MRI of spine: see figure.

Question: What is the diagnosis?

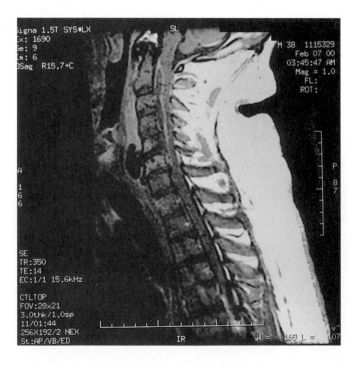

Diagnosis: Epidural/retropharyngeal abscess.

Discussion: An epidural abscess is a medical emergency. This abcess is difficult to diagnose and is often missed, as was the case for our patient. In this man, slow, progressive weakness developed over a 2-week period, with signs of a myelopathy (weakness of the right and left shoulder). He delayed returning to see his local physician because he had been started on antibiotics and was waiting for them to work. In the meantime his condition progressed to the point where his arms and legs became weak and he required an ambulance to transport him to the hospital.

The predisposing clinical settings for an epidural abscess are **furunculosis of the back or scalp**, **bacteremia**, or **minor back injury**. It can occur as a complication of local operation or, rarely, after lumbar puncture. Spinal osteomyelitis acts as the nidus for formation of an abscess that subsequently enlarges to compress the cord. There are no biological barriers in the epidural space, and the infection frequently spans three to five vertebral segments, with the potential to cover the entire spinal canal. Radiographs of the spine often are not helpful. MRI is the best diagnostic tool to find an epidural abscess if one is suspected.

The usual course is unexplained fever and mild spinal ache with local tenderness; radicular pain occurs later. When the abscess expands, it rapidly causes cord compression with symptoms of myelopathy. Treatment is **laminectomy** with drainage of the abscess and decompression, followed by appropriate antibiotics. *Staphylcoccal aureus* is seen in 60–90% of cases; aerobic or anaerobic streptococci are seen in 18%; and gram-negative infections are seen in 13%. Incomplete drainage is not uncommon, with formation of chronic granulomatous and fibrous reaction, which continues to compress the spinal cord. The likelihood of good neurologic recovery is dismal if surgery is delayed for longer than 24 hours after onset of paralysis. Other unfavorable prognostic indicators are advanced age (> 60 years); substantial thecal sac compression on imagery; and longer duration of symptom development. The prognosis for an individual with an epidural abscess is: 40% recover completely, 25% have residual weakness, 20% have permanent paralysis, and 15% die.

In the present patient, the epidural abscess was clearly visible on MRI (see figure). His condition deteriorated rapidly. He underwent emergent laminectomy with abscess drainage and irrigation. Purulent material was encountered anteriorly in the longus colli muscles; within the C5–6 vertebral disc; and posterior to the posterior longitudinal ligament. The entire C5–6 vertebral disc was involved, and partial corpectomies from C2 to C6 were performed to remove all of the infected material. Allograft bone was used from C2 to C6, with anterior fixation and cervical plate fixation. The postoperative course was very difficult, as acute respiratory distress syndrome developed, requiring ventilatory support and a percutaneous gastrostomy tube for nutrition. The patient eventually regained some upper and lower extremity function. On discharge from rehabilitation, he was able to stand briefly and was learning to take steps with a walker.

Clinical Pearls

1. Epidural abscess is difficult to diagnose. It should be in the differential diagnosis of anyone with fever of unknown origin and neck pain or a back ache.

2. MRI is the best diagnostic tool to detect a suspected epidural abscess.

3. Early and aggressive surgical treatment improves the prognosis in an individual with an epidural abscess.

4. Treatment consists of emergent laminectomy and evacuation of the abscess, followed by appropriate antibiotics.

REFERENCES

1. Hirschmann JV: Bacterial infections of the CNS. In Dale DC, Federman DD (eds): Scientific American Medicine. New York, Scientific American, May 1999.
2. Ropper AH, Martin JB: Diseases of the spinal cord. In Wilson JD, et al. (eds):Harrison's Principles of Internal Medicine, 12th ed. New York, McGraw-Hill, 1991.
3. Wood GW II: Infections of the spine. In Canale ST (ed): Campbell's Operative Orthopaedics. New York, Mosby, 1998, pp 3102–3103.

PATIENT 34

A 30-year-old man with progressive back pain and stiffness

A 30-year-old grocery store clerk presents to a spine clinic with a several-year history of progressive back stiffness and intermittent episodes of back and bilateral buttock pain. His symptoms are worse upon waking and gradually improve during the day. He denies any radiation of symptoms to the lower extremities. He is otherwise in good health and does not take any medications. He has previously received physical therapy, but admits to performing his home exercises infrequently.

Physical Examination: Vital signs: normal. Neurologic: strength and sensation normal in upper and lower extremities; deep tendon reflexes 2+ bilaterally. Musculoskeletal: thoracic kyphotic posture; on Schober's test, 1.5 cm difference between standing and flexion; bilateral SI joints tender; straight leg raise limited to 60° due to hamstring tightness, but does not produce radicular pain; mild restriction in hip internal and external rotation; extremities/joints otherwise normal. Cardiac: normal. Chest: normal expansion. HEENT: normal.

Laboratory Findings: Plain radiographs of lumbosacral spine (see figures): flattening of normal lumbar lordotic curve; anterior squaring of lumbar vertebral bodies; sacroiliac joints sclerotic; ischial tuberosities blurred.

Questions: What is the diagnosis? How would you manage this patient?

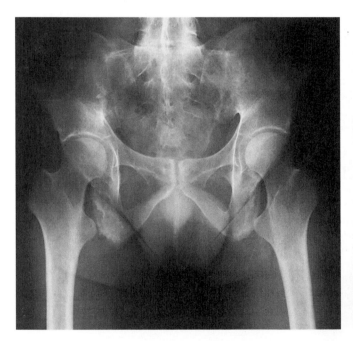
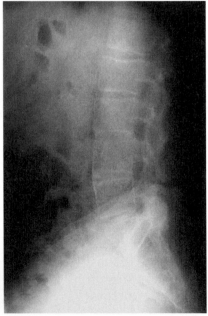

Diagnosis: Ankylosing spondylitis

Discussion: Ankylosing spondylitis (AS) is a chronic inflammatory disease that affects primarily the axial skeleton. It affects men three times more commonly than women, typically with onset during late adolescence or early adulthood. Its association with the HLA-B27 antigen is well established, although the pathogenesis and etiology of the disease is not well understood. Caucasians express the HLA-B27 antigen more frequently than other populations, and have a higher incidence of the disease. Japanese and people of African descent rarely develop the disease. The **characteristic pathologic features** of AS are inflammation of joints and insertions of joint capsules and ligaments to bone (entheses). This results in bony erosion, osseous proliferation, and ,eventually, fusion of the joints (ankylosis).

The typical presentation is insidious onset of back pain persisting for at least 3 months. Morning stiffness and improvement with exercise should alert the physician to the possibility of inflammatory disease. More than one-third of patients have symptoms affecting the appendicular skeleton. The hip is the most common peripheral joint involved, although the shoulder, knee, wrist, and metacarpophalangeal and metatarsophalangeal joints may be affected as well. Enthesopathy may affect the ischial tuberosities, iliac crests, epicondyles of the elbows, shoulders, and insertions of the plantar fascia and Achilles tendon. Acute anterior uveitis occurs in 20–30% of patients and is the most common extraskeletal manifestation. Cardiac and pulmonary involvement is rare and typically occurs late in the course of the disease.

Laboratory studies are not necessary for the diagnosis to be made. Erythrocyte sedimentation rate and C-reactive protein are commonly elevated, particularly during active phases of the disease and when peripheral joints are involved. HLA-B27 antigen testing is generally unnecessary, unless the diagnosis is uncertain based on clinical and radiologic factors. **Schober's test**, which measures lumbar spine flexion, is helpful: with the patient standing upright, a midline mark is placed at the level of the posterior superior iliac spine, as well as 10 cm above and 5 cm below. The patient is instructed to bend forward with the knees straight, and the distance between the superior and inferior marks is remeasured. Normally, it increases by at least 5 cm; an increase less than 4 cm is considered abnormal.

The clinical course of AS is variable, but characterized by exacerbations and remissions. In most patients, disability is minimal. Factors that may lead to significant disability include hip joint pathology, severe disease during the first 10 years after onset, and complete ankylosis of the cervical spine along with kyphotic deformity. The disease progresses in a caudal to cephalad stepwise fashion, with the sacroiliac joints (SIJ) affected first. **Sacroiliitis** is considered the hallmark finding of AS. It occurs early in nearly all patients. Its presence is required for the diagnosis to be made by most standard criteria. SIJ involvement is symmetric and affects the cartilaginous distal two-thirds of the joint on the iliac side.

The vertebral bodies are affected early in the disease, as well. Bony erosion at the attachment of the annulus fibrosus to the endplates leads to anterior squaring of vertebral bodies, and sclerosis at the insertions results in the "shiny corners" seen radiographically. As the disease progresses, syndesmophytes result from ossification of the outer fibers of the annulus fibrosus. They are oriented vertically and eventually bridge the intervertebral space. Over time, additional involvement of zygapophyseal joints and supraspinous and interspinous ligaments leads to the classic **bamboo spine** seen in late AS. Once ankylosis involves the cervical spine, fracture may occur with minor trauma, most commonly at C5-6 or C6-7. Spontaneous atlantoaxial subluxation occurs in 2% of patients.

Treatment is directed at preventing deformity, preserving function, and treating inflammation. Early education is important. The patient should be instructed to walk erect, sleep prone or supine on a firm mattress without a pillow, and avoid sleeping in a curled up position. Physical therapy and exercise should emphasize back extensor muscle strengthening, maintenance of flexibility in the spine, lower extremities, shoulders, and thoracic cage. Deep breathing exercises will help preserve expansion. Swimming should be advocated. Exercises requiring prolonged flexion, such as bicycling, should be avoided. Aside from exercise, nonsteroidal anti-inflammatory medications are the cornerstone of treatment. Indomethacin is the most commonly used, although GI side effects are a concern. Severe spinal deformity may require surgical intervention. Total hip replacement may be necessary with severe hip pathology.

Clinical Pearls

1. Ankylosing spondylitis presents insidiously in young patients with back pain and stiffness that improves with activity.

2. Sacroiliitis is an early finding in nearly all patients, occurs bilaterally, and is characterized radiographically by blurring of the subchondral bone, followed by erosion and sclerosis.

3. Syndesmophytes result from ossification of the outer fibers of the annulus fibrosus. They are oriented vertically and, as the disease advances, bridge the intervertebral space, leading to the classic "bamboo spine."

4. Education is the primary management for patients to prevent deformity and maintain good posture and chest expansion. Patients are taught to do back extension exercises daily, walk erect, sleep prone or supine (not curled on their side), use a firm mattress with no pillow, and avoid flexion activities such as bike riding.

REFERENCES

1. Benoist M: Inflammatory disorders. In Wiesel SW, et al (eds): The Lumbar Spine (Vol 2). The International Society for the Study of the Lumbar Spine. Philadelphia, Saunders, 1995, pp 797–811.
2. Bessette L, Katz JN, Liang MH: Differential diagnosis and conservative treatment of rheumatic disorders. In Frymoyer JW (ed): The Adult Spine, 2nd ed. Philadelphia, Lippincott-Raven, 1997, pp 803–811.
3. Schumacher HR, Klippel JH, Koopman WJ: Seronegative spondylarthropathies: Ankylosing spondylitis. In: Primer on rheumatic diseases, 11th ed. Atlanta, GA, Arthritis Foundation, 1993, pp 180–183.

PATIENT 35

A 25-year-old man with right knee pain, intermittent swelling, and instability

A 25-year-old man presents with a 1-year history of right knee pain, intermittent swelling, and a feeling of "giving away." He is a very athletic individual and recalls a football injury about 1 year ago. He has continued to play football and other contact sports, but the symptoms have become more frequent, and even minor tackles with his right leg planted give him trouble. The knee has never locked. There is no numbness, tingling, or weakness, and no history of hip or back pain. He has no significant past medical or surgical history.

Physical Examination: Gait: mildly antalgic. Musculoskeletal: minimal right knee effusion; minimal medial joint line tenderness and patellofemoral tenderness; no quadriceps atrophy; McMurray's test positive; positive Lachman's test and anterior drawer sign; collateral ligaments and posterior drawer tests negative. The patient would not allow a pivot shift test. Range of motion: 0–130 degrees, but pain at end range. Neurologic and vascular: normal.

Laboratory Findings: X-ray of right knee: normal.

Questions: What is the clinical diagnosis? How would you proceed?

Answers: The diagnosis is torn anterior cruciate ligament and a probable tear of medial meniscus in right knee. Additional imaging studies, such as an MRI, should be performed to confirm the clinical diagnosis and help plan further management

Discussion: Anterior cruciate ligament (ACL) injury is quite common: approximately 80,000 occur annually in the United States. The highest incidence is in individuals 15–25 years old who participate in pivoting sports. The estimated cost for these injuries is almost a billion dollars per year.

Seventy percent of ACL injuries occur in non-contact situations. Noncontact mechanisms are classified as sudden deceleration prior to a change of direction or landing motion. Contact injuries occur as a result of valgus collapse of the knee. The risk factors for non-contact ACL injuries fall into four categories: environmental, anatomic, hormonal, and biomechanical.

The history and physical examination are by far the most important means of diagnosis. Arthrometeric measurement with comparison to the normal side adds to the quantification of laxity. MRI is required in most cases to confirm the clinical diagnosis and to assess the status of the menisci and collateral ligaments.

Management depends on the patient's personal choice, activity level, current function, and type of meniscal injury. Conservative treatment may be offered to a less active and less physically demanding individual who has an isolated ACL injury. An aggressive rehabilitation program and bracing is recommended. Braces can decrease anterior tibial translation 28.8% to 39.1% without the stabilizing contractions of the hamstring, quadriceps, and gastrocnemius muscles. With lower extremity muscle activation and bracing, anterior tibial translation can be decreased 69.8% to 84.9%. Laterally hinged braces are as effective as the more commonly used double-hinged models.

Surgical management is recommended for more active patients. Patients managed nonsurgically may complain of instability: there is an increased incidence of meniscal tears and degenerative arthritis in nonsurgically managed patients. Age does not appear to disqualify middle-aged patients with symptomatic ACL tears from undergoing reconstruction. Factors such as mental preparation of the patient; school, work, family, and social schedules; and preoperative condition of the knee (e.g., minimal or no swelling, good strength, good leg control, and full range of motion) must be considered before undertaking surgery.

Surgical management of the ACL-deficient knee has evolved from primary repair to extracapsular augmentation to anterior cruciate ligament reconstruction using biologic tissue grafts. Currently, harvesting the central third of the patellar tendon for autograft ACL reconstruction is considered a gold standard. It does not diminish quadriceps strength or functional capacity in highly active patients who receive intensive rehabilitation. Allograft use has also been recommended with good success.

Arthrofibrosis is a potential complication of acute ACL reconstruction. Arthrofibrosis prevents the patient from regaining full range of motion, particularly the terminal 5 degrees of full extension, postoperatively. Arthrofibrosis is more likely to develop in patients whose ligaments are reconstructed within the first week after injury than in patients for whom ACL reconstruction is delayed 21 days or more.

A wide spectrum of protocols are available for rehabilitation after ACL reconstruction. The strengthening program should emphasize closed rather than open kinetic chain exercises. Later, neuromuscular-proprioceptive training and sport-specific agility training may be needed to redevelop reaction time for athletes. Use of continuous passive motion does not effect long-term results. An accelerated rehabilitation program after ACL reconstruction also does not affect long-term stability of the graft as measured by the KT-1000 arthrometer.

In the present patient, MRI (see figure) revealed an ACL tear—probably from his first injury about 1 year ago. Arthroscopic examination revealed complex tears of medial and lateral menisci, most likely due to his continued activity after the initial injury. He required an autograft of the central third of the patellar tendon for ACL reconstruction, and excision of the irreparable torn pieces of the medial and lateral menisci. He participated in an accelerated rehabilitation program with good results at follow-up.

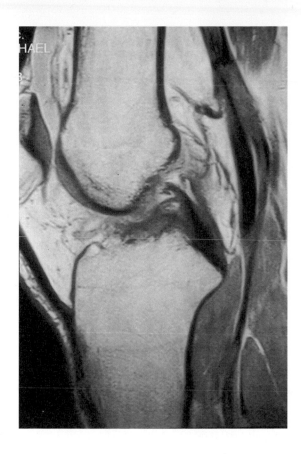

Clinical Pearls

1. Seventy percent of ACL injuries occur in noncontact situations.

2. History and physical examination are >95% diagnostic. Two-thirds of patients managed by nonoperative means complain of instability.

3. Laterally hinged braces are as effective as the more commonly used double-hinged models.

4. Closed kinetic chain exercises after ACL reconstruction cause less patellofemoral pain, and patients are generally more satisfied with the end result, returning to normal daily activities and sports sooner than expected.

REFERENCES

1. Bynum EB, Barrack RL, Alexander AH: Open versus closed chain kinetic exercises after anterior cruciate ligament reconstruction. A prospective randomized study. Am J Sports Med 23:401–406, 1995.
2. Fu FH, Bennett CH, Ma CB, et al: Current trends in anterior cruciate ligament reconstruction. Part II. Operative procedures and clinical correlations. Am J Sports Med 28:124–130, 2000.
3. Griffin LY, Agel J, Albohm MJ, et al: Noncontact anterior cruciate ligament injuries: Risk factors and prevention strategies: J Am Acad Orthop Surg 8:141–150, 2000.
4. Shelbourne KD, Patel DV: Timing of surgery in anterior cruciate ligament-injured knees. Knee Surg Sports Traumatol Arthrosc 3:148–156, 1995.
5. Wojtys EM, Kothari SU, Huston LJ: Anterior cruciate ligament functional brace use in sports. Am J Sports Med 24:539–546, 1996.

PATIENT 36

A 68-year-old woman with a history of obesity and right knee pain

A 68-year-old woman presented with right knee pain. She was employed in a manufacturing plant, and her job required lifting boxes weighing up to 70 pounds multiple times per day. After retiring, the patient began experiencing difficulty walking due to pain in her knees. The right knee pain had progressed over the past 6 months and occurred at rest and when she was trying to sleep. Her treatment included acetaminophen, NSAIDs, physical therapy, exercises, viscosupplementation, and multiple injections of steroids into the knee joint. The patient had little response to conservative treatment; therefore, she was recommended for total knee replacement by her orthopedist. She underwent surgery approximately 1 week ago and has now been transferred to acute inpatient rehabilitation.

She was recently diagnosed with atrial fibrillation and placed on Coumadin. Past medical history also includes obesity since adolescence, hypertension, congestive heart failure, and diabetes mellitus. She is taking Lotensin and insulin in addition to Coumadin. Family history reveals obesity, diabetes mellitus in her mother and maternal grandmother, and arthritis in her grandmother.

Physical Examination: General: morbidly obese, no apparent distress. Cardiac: irregularly irregular. Chest: clear to auscultation. Musculoskeletal: severe valgus deformity in left knee in stance phase of gait; large anterior surgical incision with staples in right knee; passive range of motion markedly limited (−5 extension to 40 degrees flexion); moderate swelling of knee; no calf tenderness or swelling.

Laboratory Findings: Rheumatoid factor, ANA, ESR: negative. Radiographs: right knee— good alignment of total knee prosthesis, mild soft tissue swelling; left knee—moderate medial and lateral compartment narrowing, periarticular osteophytes.

Questions: What is the hallmark of osteoarthritis? What is the mainstay of treatment in the acute rehabilitation phase of total knee arthroplasty?

Answers: Cartilage degeneration. Continuous passive range of motion is the mainstay of treatment.

Discussion: Cartilage degeneration is the main characteristic of osteoarthritis (OA). The pathophysiology of this process involves many inflammatory mediators. Although frank inflammation is usually not seen, subclinical inflammation plays a significant role in the progression of OA. Specifically, interleukin 1, nitrous oxide, and prostaglandin appear to drive catabolic changes in the cartilage. In vitro studies have also pointed to the possibility of an interaction between subchondral bone and cartilage as a part of the disease.

The breakdown of the cartilage matrix leads to gross defects characterized by fissures. These progress into full-thickness defects leading down to subchondral bone. Bone changes include osteophyte formation and sclerosis or thickening of the subchondral bone plate. Inflammatory cytokines then mediate a catabolic process, which is first produced in the synovial membrane, then diffused in the cartilage through the synovial fluid.

Some data suggests that interleukin-1 (IL-1) and tumor necrosis factor-alpha (TNF-α) are the major players. Both of these cytokines have been found in enhanced amounts in the synovial membrane of individuals with OA. Cartilage of osteoarthritis patients also produces a large amount of nitric oxide. Current therapeutic strategies for blocking IL-1 and TNF-α have proven valuable in other arthritic diseases and in animal models. Experiments have also shown that inhibiting nitrous oxide synthase has slowed the progression of lesions in OA.

Theories regarding the role of subchondral bone in the pathophysiology of OA include healing trabecular microfractures, which result in stiffer bone that is no longer an effective shock absorber. A possible explanation for this altered bone is abnormal osteoblast behavior. This process, coupled with mechanical and chemical stresses, could accelerate subchondral bone formation, increasing the mechanical pressure on the cartilage and supporting joints.

Another clear part of the pathophysiology involves inflammatory processes that may affect the cartilage in an endocrine/paracrine fashion to upregulate matrix homeostasis. Matrix metalloproteases have potential for cartilage matrix changes that lead to osteoarthritis.

The role of COX2 in osteoarthritis synovial tissue has begun to be examined more closely with the development of selective COX2 inhibitors. These medications are widely used for their analgesic effects in OA and rheumatoid arthritis.

Total knee arthroplasty is indicated for patients who fail conservative management and continue to have significant pain that limits their functional abilities. The use of **continuous passive motion machines** (CPM) within 48 hours of replacement surgery has been shown to decrease pain and also decrease the length of hospital stay. The major problem after total knee arthroplasty is limited flexion. The main goal of CPM and passive range-of-motion exercises by a physical therapist is to achieve 90 degrees of knee flexion. In an attempt to allow proper healing, isometric exercises generally are not started until 8 weeks postoperatively. A recent study comparing home CPM use to formal inpatient therapy by physical therapists showed no advantage to inpatient therapy. However, formal therapy should be sought at least initially to ensure a proper home program.

Total knee arthroplasty components have improved over recent years and are generally thought to last for longer than 10 years. For properly selected patients, total knee arthroplasty can tremendously improve functional abilities and quality of life.

Clinical Pearls

1. Cartilage degeneration is the hallmark of osteoarthritis.
2. Inflammatory mediators play a significant role in the etiology and progression of osteoarthritis.
3. Continuous passive range of motion within 48 hours has been shown to decrease hospital stay in total knee arthroplasty.
4. The main goal of rehabilitation is improved knee flexion. Isometric exercises are initially avoided.

REFERENCES

1. Abramson SB: The role of COX-2 produced by cartilage in arthritis. Osteoarthritis Cartilage 7(4):380–381, 1999.
2. Braddom RL: Physical Medicine & Rehabilitation. Philadelphia, W.B. Saunders, 1996.
3. Martel-Pelletier J: Pathophysiology of osteoarthritis. Osteoarthritis Cartilage 6(6):374–376, 1998.
4. Rehman Q, Lane NE: Getting control of osteoarthritis pain. Postgrad Med 106(4):127–134, 1999.
5. Schwartz ST, Zimmermann B: Update on osteoarthritis. Med Health R I 82(9):321–324, 1999.

PATIENT 37

A 64-year-old man with cough and sputum production

A 64-year-old man with a 4-year history of cough with occasional sputum production presents with increasing shortness of breath and cough of 6-month duration. He quit smoking cigarettes 5 years ago, after totaling 50 pack-years. He has been on portable home oxygen at 2 liters for the past 4 months. His medications include aspirin, a bronchodilator inhaler, a steroid inhaler, theophylline, and a diuretic. His quality of life has markedly declined in the past 6 months due to his worsening respiratory status, reduced energy, and emotional decline.

Physical Examination: Temperature 99°, pulse 104, blood pressure 145/92, respirations 25 with use of accessory muscles of respiration. Cardiac: heart sounds distant, without murmur. Chest: barrel chest, hyper-resonant, crackles in bases, inspiratory wheezes, prolonged expiratory phase with grunting, no egophony. Abdomen: moderately obese, normal sounds, nontender. Extremities: clubbing of nails on hands and feet; no edema; cool distal extremities; 2+ pulses in arms, 1+ in legs.

Laboratory Findings: WBC 6200/μl, Hct 41%, platelets 352,000/μl. Arterial blood gas (2 L oxygen per nasal canula): pH 7.31 (7.35–7.45 normal), PaO$_2$ 62 mmHg (80–105 mmHg), PCO$_2$ 50 mmHg (35–45 mmHg), HCO$_3^-$ 28 mEq/L (22–26 mEq/L), O$_2$ saturation 92%. Chest x-ray (see figure): on anteroposterior view, flattening and depression of diaphragm, areas of hypertransradiancy in lung zones, and narrow cardiac shadow; on lateral view (not shown), increased retrosternal air space.

Question: Why does this patient have a prolonged expiratory phase during respiration?

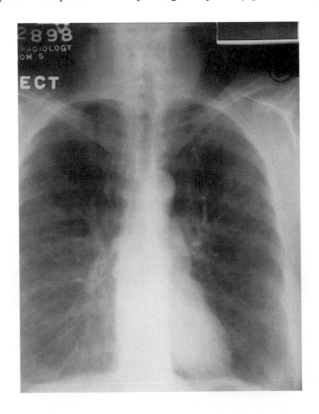

Answer: Air trapping due to chronic obstructive pulmonary disease (COPD) is causing the prolonged expiratory phase. He has emphysema with chronic bronchitis.

Discussion: COPD is an umbrella diagnosis that includes diseases such as emphysema, chronic bronchitis, chronic asthma, and chronic bronchiolitis. The main common denominators are chronicity, marked respiratory compromise, and small and/or large airway obstruction from inflammation, small airway collapse, or non-exertional airway hyper-reactivity. Periods of exacerbation from respiratory infection are common. COPD is the fifth leading cause of mortality in North America, and is rising from that position. Cigarette smoking is the greatest risk factor.

COPD is best managed using a multidisciplinary approach. **Pulmonary rehabilitation**—a team approach for treating patient with COPD—incorporates medical management, exercise reconditioning, coping skills, nutrition, nursing support, and education. Commonly applied exercises include treadmill, water therapy, ergometry, and respiratory muscle training.

Many studies have shown that pulmonary rehabilitation reduces dyspnea and hospitalization rates, lowers respiratory rates, and improves exercise tolerance. Ability to engage in activities of daily living and 12-minute timed walks also improve. While some studies reveal improvement in PaO_2, FEV1, FVC, and maximal inspiratory pressures, pulmonary rehabilitation is not believed to significantly improve pulmonary function. Other positive results include reduction in anxiety and depression and better ability to cope with the disease.

Pulmonary rehabilitation gives people with COPD an improved quality of life.

The present patient's doctor changed his metered dose albuterol inhaler to the same medicine in nebulized form, and increased the theophylline dose. The patient was enrolled in a 6-week pulmonary rehabilitation program incorporating the different interventions described above. He found the relaxation techniques and coping strategies helpful. The respiratory therapist set him up with continuous positive airway pressure for nocturnal use; his ABG showed the common situation of chronic respiratory acidosis partially compensated by the kidneys via reduction of bicarbonate excretion, as seen in COPD. The respiratory therapist instructed him on suctioning, pursed-lip breathing, and exercises such as chest expansion and inspiratory resistance training. The therapist also taught his wife to perform chest percussion to help loosen the secretions.

A dietician formulated a low-carbohydrate diet to lower his carbon dioxide production, and he was instructed to increase his water intake. Proper nutrition to improve respiratory muscle function and immune defenses is vital for people with COPD; yet, surprisingly, up to 50% of inpatients with COPD are malnourished. The present patient's nurse educated him on avoiding smoking and environmental pulmonary irritants, medication usage, and infection and signs of exacerbation. The present patient's quality of life greatly improved following the pulmonary rehabilitation program.

Clinical Pearls

1. COPD is the fifth leading cause of mortality in North America.

2. Pulmonary rehabilitation reduces respiration rates, length of hospital stays, anxiety, and depression. It improves exercise tolerance, ability to engage in activities of daily living, timed 12-minute walk, and coping ability.

3. Pulmonary rehabilitation is not generally believed to significantly improve pulmonary function.

4. Proper nutrition is vital for people with COPD because it improves respiratory muscle function and immune defenses. Nevertheless, approximately 50% of inpatients with COPD are malnourished.

REFERENCES
1. Alba AS: Concepts in pulmonary rehabilitation. In Braddom RL (ed): Physical Medicine and Rehabilitation. Philadelphia, WB Saunders, 1996, pp 671–685.
2. Bach JR, Moldover JR: Cardiovascular, pulmonary, and cancer rehabilitation. 2. Pulmonary rehabilitation. Arch Phys Med Rehabil 77:S45–S51, 1996.
3. Lacasse Y, Wong E, Guyatt GH, et al: Meta-analysis of respiratory rehabilitation in chronic obstructive pulmonary disease. Lancet 348(9035):1115–1119, 1996.
4. Thomas CL: Taber's Cyclopedic Medical Dictionary, 18th ed. Philadelphia, FA Davis Company, 1997.

PATIENT 38

A 51-year-old man with mid to low back pain, malaise, and excessive thirst

A 51-year-old man presents with back pain of 4-month duration. He states that the pain is "band-like" and generalizes to the mid and low back region, is worse at night while lying in the supine position, and is not relieved with ibuprofen, acetaminophen, or rest. Previous plain films of the lumbar and thoracic spine showed osteopenia, but otherwise were unrevealing. Pain has been steadily getting worse in intensity despite physical therapy— intense enough to frequently awaken him from sleep. Review of systems reveals an occasional low-grade fever and a general feeling of malaise accompanied by excessive thirst.

Physical Examination: General well-nourished; no distress aside from back pain. Chest: clear to auscultation. Abdomen: soft, nontender. Musculoskeletal: mild, diffuse tenderness along both thoracic paraspinal muscles; straight-leg raising negative. Neurologic: intact and otherwise normal.

Laboratory Findings: Hemoglobin 5.2 g/dl, WBC 4700/µl, platelets 185,000/µl, reticulocytes 0.9%. Creatinine 5.4 mg/dl, clearance 18.1 ml/min; electrolytes normal; calcium 14.4 mg/dl. X-ray of head: see figure.

Questions: What is the significance of this patient's symptoms? What other imaging or laboratory studies might be helpful?

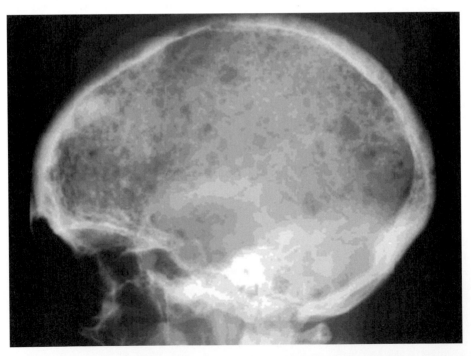

From Soutar R: Multiple myeloma: Clinical aspects of bone disease. Proceedings (30)1, 1998; with permission.

Answers: This patient's age and symptoms suggest multiple myeloma. The confirmatory lab test is 24-hour urinalysis by protein electrophoresis to determine the presence of monoclonal Bence Jones proteins.

Discussion: Two thirds of patients with multiple myeloma complain of bone pain, frequently located in the back, long bones, skull, and pelvis. The most common presentation is low back pain. Multiple myeloma is the malignant proliferation of plasma cells involving more than 10% of the bone marrow. As a result, osteoblastic activity is inhibited, and osteoclast-activating factors are produced, causing painful lytic lesions and hypercalcemia. These malignant cells also produce monoclonal immunoglobulins that may be identified on serum or urine protein electrophoresis. Thus, all patients with suspected multiple myeloma should have a 24-hour urinalysis by protein electrophoresis to determine the presence of monoclonal Bence Jones proteins.

The differential diagnosis of multiple myeloma includes monoclonal gammopathy, heavy chain disease, plasmacytoma, and Waldenstrom macroglobulinemia. Treatment includes chemotherapy with melphalan-prednisone, combination chemotherapy, alfa interferon, and stem-cell marrow transplantation. Multiple myeloma should be considered as a diagnosis in patients over 50 years of age with back pain persisting more than 1 month if one or more of the following characteristics of pain are identified:
- Worse in the supine position
- Worse at night or awakens patient from sleep
- A band-like distribution around the body
- Not relieved with conventional methods
- Associated constitutional symptoms (fever, weight loss, dehydration).

In the present patient, the skull radiograph revealed numerous punched-out lytic lesions, consistent with multiple myeloma. While such osteolytic lesions may be observed in the lumbar or thoracic spine, this case illustrates that osteopenia may be the only identifiable abnormality seen in spine films; hence the need for additional imaging and laboratory studies to make the diagnosis. Subsequent 24-hour urinalysis by protein electrophoresis demonstrated the presence of monoclonal Bence Jones proteins.

Clinical Pearls

1. Early in the disease, lytic lesions from multiple myeloma may be difficult to see on plain radiographs of the lumbar spine.
2. Excessive thirst may be a symptom of hypercalcemia due to multiple myeloma.

REFERENCES
1. Burton CH, Fairham SA, Millet B, et al: Unusual aetiology of persistent back pain in a patient with multiple myeloma: Infectious discitis. J Clin Pathol 51:633–634, 1998.
2. Chukwudelunzu FE, Meschia JF: A 49-year-old woman with back pain and loss of consciousness. Mayo Clin Proc 73:687–690, 1998.
3. Rabb H, Gunasekaran H, Gunasekaran S, Saba SR: Acute renal failure from multiple myeloma precipitated by ACE inhibitors. Am J Kidney Dis 33:E5, 1999
4. George ED, Sadovsky R: Multiple myeloma: Recognition and management. Am Fam Physician 59:1885–1894, 1999.
5. Davies FE, Anderson KC: Novel therapeutic targets in multiple myeloma. Eur J Haematol 64:359–367, 2000.
6. Kanis JA, McCloskey EV: Bisphosphonates in multiple myeloma. Cancer 88:3022–3032, 2000.

PATIENT 39

A 60-year-old man with left hand weakness

A 60-year-old man is referred from a primary care clinic for evaluation of left hand weakness. One year ago, he fell and dislocated his left shoulder. He waited 3 days after the fall before he sought medical attention. He noticed weakness of his left arm immediately after the accident, but believed that his strength was improving. His presenting complaint is of continuing difficulty using his left hand.

Physical Examination: General: left claw hand. Musculoskeletal: manual muscle testing intact throughout right upper extremity; in left upper extremity, shoulder abduction 2/5, shoulder internal rotation 4/5, shoulder external rotation 2/5, elbow extension and flexion, wrist extension 5/5, abductor pollicis brevis 3/5, abductor digite quinte 2/5. Neurologic: light touch appreciation decreased in left C6-C8 dermatomes, but intact in right upper extremity; biceps, brachioradialis, and triceps reflexes decreased but symmetric in both upper extremities.

Laboratory Findings: See results of nerve conduction and EMG studies below.

Question: What is causing these left hand problems?

Nerve Conduction Study

Nerve	Site	Latency	CV	Amplitude
L ulnar (motor)	Wrist-ADQ	4.1 ms		1.0 mV
	Elbow-wrist		45 m/s	0.8 mV
L ulnar (sensory)	Wrist-digit V	NR		
L dorsal ulnar cutaneous (sens)	Wrist-dorsal hand	NR		
L radial (sensory)	Wrist-digit I	NR		
L med antebrach cutaneous	Forearm-elbow	NR		
R ulnar (sensory)	Wrist-digit V	3.7 msec	37.8 m/s	10 µV
R dorsal ulnar cutaneous	Wrist-dorsal hand	NR		
R ulnar (motor)	Wrist-ADQ	2.9 msec		3.5 mV
	Elbow-wrist		55 m/s	3.1 mV
R radial (sensory)	Wrist-digit I	2.7 msec	37 m/s	5 µV

CV = conduction velocity, ADQ = abductor digite quinte, NR = no response

EMG Study

Muscle	Insertional Activity	MUAP Morphology	MUAP Recruitment
L lateral deltoid	2+fibs/PSW - 100–200 µV	Polyphasic	Few MUAP seen
L posterior deltoid	Normal	Normal	Normal
L biceps	Normal	Normal	Normal
L triceps	Normal	Normal	Normal
L pronator teres	Occas PSW	Normal	Normal
L flexor pollicus longus	2+ fibs/PSW 50–150 µV	50% polyphasic	Normal
L flexor carpi ulnaris	3+PSW, 1+fibs 100-200 µV	30% polyphasics with inc. amplitude	Moderate dropout
L teres minor	Occas PSW	30% polyphasic	Normal
L teres major	Normal	Normal	Normal
L infraspinatous	Normal	Normal	Normal
L cervical paraspinals	Normal	—	—

MUAP = motor unit action potential, PSW = positive sharp waves

Diagnosis: Traumatic brachial plexopathy affecting the medial cord and anterior branch of the axillary nerve

Discussion: The brachial plexus is formed from five spinal nerve roots (C5 through T1). It supplies most of the sensory, motor, and sympathetic nerve fibers to the upper limb. The roots divide into the dorsal and ventral rami, with only the ventral rami contributing to the brachial plexus. The ventral rami of C5 and C6 unite to form the upper trunk, C7 continues as the middle trunk, and C8 and T1 unite to form the lower trunk. Each trunk then divides into anterior and posterior divisions. The anterior divisions form the medial and lateral cords. The three posterior divisions unite to form the posterior cord. The peripheral nerves of the upper limb are branches of these cords.

The brachial plexus passes over the first rib behind the middle third of the clavicle to enter the axilla. The roots and trunks are proximal to the clavicle. Beneath the clavicle are the divisions, and distal to the clavicle are the cords and terminal branches. The etiology of brachial plexus injuries includes trauma, neoplastic infiltration (especially lung, breast, lymphomas), radiation treatment, and idiopathic (Parsonage-Turner syndrome).

The preferred method for making a diagnosis of brachial plexus injury, especially for determination of the extent of the injury and the prognosis, remains electrodiagnostic studies. Results from the electrodiagnostic testing vary according to the type of injury. With denervating injuries, electromyographic evidence of denervation and/or reinnervation should be present in more than a single root or peripheral nerve distribution, and the paraspinal musculature should be spared. Plexopathies due to conduction block may be difficult to demonstrate with electrodiagnostic testing.

Sensory nerve action potentials (SNAPs) should be affected if the lesion is postganglionic, and spared if preganglionic. If the sensory nerve is severed, the SNAPs may be normal for 3–5 days, after which the amplitude will gradually decrease, then disappear in 7-10 days. Distal latencies and nerve conduction velocities (NCV) may be normal if fast conducting sensory fibers are spared. If the plexopathy is due only to a conduction block, the SNAPs should recover quickly. Mild, partial lesions may not affect sensory amplitude. Because of variations of amplitudes in normal individuals and the possibility that only one side is affected by the plexopathy, sensory studies should be performed on the patient's unaffected side to detect an abnormal SNAP by comparison.

Compound motor action potential (CMAPs) amplitude is a more important parameter than distal latencies and NCV. As is the case with sensory nerve studies, if the fast fibers are spared and the lesion is incomplete, latencies and NCV may not be affected distal to the lesion. Side-to-side comparison is recommended in such cases. If the plexopathy results in axonal loss, CMAP amplitude should begin to decrease after 5–10 days due to Wallerian degeneration. If CMAP amplitude does not decrease, the electromyographer should suspect that the weakness is due to a conduction block, which has a better prognosis for recovery. For both the motor and sensory nerve conduction studies, the electromyographer needs to know the appropriate sensory and motor nerve for each level of brachial plexus (see tables on next page).

This patient had evidence of a post-ganglionic lesion because SNAPs were absent on the affected side. The decreased amplitude of the CMAPs on the affected side and the evidence of denervation and reinnervation on needle exam were indicative of axonal loss. The denervation and reinnervation changes were seen in muscles from multiple root levels and with common innervation from the medial cord. The exceptions to this common innervation were the posterior deltoid and teres minor muscles, which are both innervated from the posterior branch of the axillary nerve and the posterior cord.

Suspected brachial plexopathies need to be differentiated from single- or multiple-level radiculopathies. Prognosis depends on the underlying cause and severity of the initial lesion.

Sensory Nerve Conduction Study

Trunk	Cord	Peripheral Nerve
Upper	Lateral	Lateral antebrachial cutaneous
Upper	Lateral	Median to digit I and II
Upper	Posterior	Radial to digit I
Middle	Posterior	Posterior antebrachial cutaneous
Middle	Lateral	Median to digit II
Middle	Lateral	Median to digit III
Lower	Medial	Ulnar to digit V
Lower	Medial	Dorsal ulnar cutaneous
Lower	Medial	Medial antebrachial cutaneous

Motor Nerve Conduction Study

Trunk	Cord	Peripheral Nerve
Upper	Lateral	Musculocutaneous
Upper	Posterior	Axillary
Upper	—	Suprascapular
Middle	Posterior	Radial
Lower	Medial	Median
Lower	Medial	Ulnar

Both tables are from Dumitru D: Brachial plexopathies and proximal mononeuropathies. In Dumitru D (ed): Electrodiagnostic Medicine. Philadelphia, Hanley & Belfus, 1995, p 598; with permission.

Clinical Pearls

1. The electromyographer should know the appropriate sensory and motor nerve for each level of the brachial plexus.

2. Patients are their own best controls for normal values; therefore, compare NCS of the affected side with the unaffected side.

3. Typically, SNAPs are affected if the lesion is postganglionic, and spared if the lesion is preganglionic. However, CMAPs may be affected by both preganglionic and postganglionic lesions.

4. Plexopathies due to conduction block may be difficult to demonstrate with electrodiagnostic testing. Therefore, if the clinical findings are more severe than the findings on the electrodiagnostic examination, suspect neuropraxic lesions.

5. Lack of abnormalities on the needle examination of the paraspinal muscles supports the diagnosis of a plexopathy rather than a radiculopathy.

REFERENCES

1. Dumitru D: Brachial plexopathies and proximal mononeuropathies. In Dumitru D (ed): Electrodiagnostic Medicine. Philadelphia, Hanley & Belfus, 1995, pp 585–642.
2. Goldstein B.: Applied anatomy and electrodiagnosis of brachial plexopathies. North Am Clin Phys Med Rehabil 5:477–493, 1994.
3. Subramony SH: AAEE case report # 14: Neuralgic amyotrophy (acute brachial neuropathy). Muscle Nerve 11:39–44, 1988.

PATIENT 40

A 71-year-old man with a thrombotic stroke, left hemiplegia, and daytime sleepiness

A 71-year-old man is admitted to a rehabilitation unit after he sustained left hemiplegia from a thrombotic stroke. The initial CT scan of his head shows a small infarct in the right internal capsule, but no hemorrhage. He is frequently sleepy during his therapy sessions. The nurses report no agitation or unusual behavior during the night, except for intermittent loud snoring, which his family say is typical for the patient. He has no history of dementia or lung disease. He has not smoked nor taken any alcohol for the last 20 years.

Physical Examination: Blood pressure 155/80, pulse 79, respiration 18, temperature 98.9°. General: alert, obese (height 5 feet 10 inches, weight 270 pounds). Cardiac: regular rate and rhythm. Chest: clear. Abdomen: flabby, soft, nontender, with normal bowel sounds. Extremities: mild left pedal edema; no warmth or redness. Neurologic: oriented to self, person, and place; speech clear and fluent; cranial nerves grossly intact except for mild left central facial weakness; sensation intact to pinprick and light touch. Musculoskeletal: 3–4/5 strength in left upper and lower extremities, 5/5 in right upper and lower extremities; muscle stretch reflexes increased on left.

Laboratory Findings: CBC, electrolytes, BUN, creatinine, glucose, and liver function tests: normal. Total cholesterol: slightly elevated at 215. HDL, LDL, and triglycerides: normal. Repeat CT of head: interval decrease in size of infarct. Chest x-ray: no acute or chronic process; heart size normal.

Question: What diagnostic test or procedure should be requested next to ascertain the reason for this patient's sleepiness?

Answer: Polysomnographic (sleep) studies, to check for sleep apnea

Discussion: Sleep apnea is found in 55–70% of patients with acute stroke or transient ischemic attacks. It is a strong risk factor for the development of a stroke episode. More than 50% of patients who have had a stroke give a history of a premorbid sleep disorder or sleep apnea. Patients with severe snoring have a 2.8 times higher risk of suffering a stroke. Clinically apparent sleep apnea is manifested by daytime sleepiness, habitual snoring, episodes of apnea and hypopnea, or oxygen desaturation below 85% during sleep. Treatment of this disorder can decrease the risk of stroke.

Obstructive sleep apnea in obese individuals is due to increased pharyngeal resistance and reduced airway patency. Hypopharyngeal collapse can occur, as well as failure of the reflex activation of airway dilator muscles. In addition, decreased total respiratory compliance in the recumbent position can be a contributing factor.

Sleep apnea may also be a result of the stroke itself (central sleep apnea). Mohsenin found that 8 out of 10 patients without a premorbid history had evidence of apnea based on sleep studies.

Diagnosis of sleep apnea is done by all-night continuous testing with full-channel polysomnography, partial polysomnography, or oxymetry measurements of oxygen saturation.

Initial measures for treatment are avoidance of the supine position, weight reduction, and use of nasal or mask CPAP (continuous positive airway pressure). Avoidance of the supine position can be done by sewing a tennis ball to the back of the patient's shirt. Weight reduction in obese patients can improve or resolve sleep apnea, but this is often temporary. CPAP is usually the next measure taken; however, the compliance rate for CPAP is low (35–50%) due to discomfort. In addition, it is not adequate for patients with restricted lung volumes and hypercapnia. BiPAP (bilevel positive airway pressure) machines can deliver independently varying inspiratory and expiratory positive airway pressures, which is more effective and comfortable.

Some patients benefit from long-term use of an orthodontic device, which helps to keep the hypopharynx open. Nasopharyngeal and tracheostomy tubes should be considered only as a last resort. Surgical procedures such as uvulopalatopharyngoplasty and advancement of the mandible, maxilla, and hyoid have been done in the past, but found ineffective.

Clinical Pearls

1. In patients with strokes or transient ischemic attacks, inquire about a history of any sleep disorder or sleep apnea.

2. Patients with a history of sleep apnea have a 2.8 times higher risk of experiencing stroke, and treatment of sleep apnea reduces the risk of stroke.

3. Sleep apnea in patients with stroke can be obstructive and/or central in origin.

4. All nonsurgical measures to treat sleep apnea should be attempted first.

REFERENCES
1. Black-Schaffer RM, Kirsteins AE, Harvey RL: Stroke rehabilitation. 2. Comorbidities and complications. Arch Phys Med Rehabil 80:S8–S16, 1999.
2. Buskirk ER: Obesity and weight control. In Downey JA, et al (eds): The Physiological Basis of Rehabilitation Medicine, 2nd ed. Boston, Butterworth-Heinemann, 1994, pp 4481–4499.
3. Halar EM: Management of stroke risk factors during the process of rehabilitation: Secondary stroke prevention. Phys Med Rehab Clin North Am 10(4):839–856, 1999.
4. Mohsenin V, Valor R: Sleep apnea in patients with hemispheric stroke. Arch Phys Med Rehabil 76:71–76, 1995.

PATIENT 41

A 9-year-old boy with an upper extremity limb length difference

The mother of this boy with known right hemiparetic cerebral palsy reports that she noticed a striking shortening of his affected arm compared to his "good" arm when, for the first time in years, he wore a long-sleeved dress shirt. He was born at term after prolonged labor via otherwise uncomplicated vaginal delivery. Hemiparesis was diagnosed at about 9 months of age, when a strong hand preference was noted. A CT head scan and EEG were done elsewhere at about 1 year of age; the mother states that they were normal. Thus, an intrauterine cerebrovascular accident was assumed. Heelcord lengthening was performed at age 4 with good results, and the patient uses a hinged ankle-foot orthotic. He tried various upper extremity orthotics, but rejects them all, and really has never used his right hand or arm functionally other than occasionally for stabilizing purposes. Physical but not occupational therapy is available where he lives, in a rural community.

Physical Examination: Skeletal: spine straight, hips clinically not subluxed, pelvis level in stance, no leg length discrepancy. Musculoskeletal: Achilles tendon reflexes brisk; right Babinski upgoing; left foot and ankle range normal, right lacking dorsiflexion range past neutral; minimal dysmetria and mildly impaired fine motor skill of left upper extremity; right upper extremity shows 10° elbow flexion contracture with brisk biceps and triceps reflex; wrist posture palmar flexed but rangeable to neutral, though finger flexors tighten when this is done. Shoulder somewhat stiff with increased tone; does not sublux with traction; range of motion 60% of expected. No functional grasp and release; grasp weak and release dystonic with excess wrist flexion and intrinsic minus posturing. Upper extremity length discrepancy about 2 cm—even allowing for the flexion contracture—and right hand noticeably smaller and less developed (see figure). Neurologic: letters X, A, and O traced on left palm distinguished at least 80% of time; only about 50% correct between X and O on the right; Horner syndrome absent, though there is an esophoria.

Laboratory Findings: None available.

Questions: Does the limb length difference require additional workup, such as electrodiagnostic study to confirm or rule out an undiagnosed brachial plexus palsy, or is it consistent with the diagnosis of right hemiparetic cerebral palsy? Can function be improved in his right arm and hand?

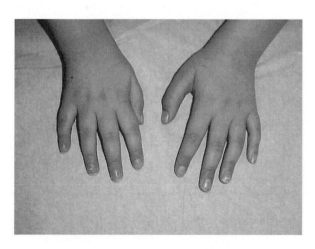

Answers: No further workup is necessary. The potential for improved function does exist.

Discussion: These symptoms are consistent with an upper motor neuron limb length discrepancy. Impaired discriminative sensation is associated with a lack of fine motor or manipulative function. More intensive, earlier therapy could have achieved better use of the extremity—at least in an assistive capacity—and prevented some contracture. There might still be potential benefit in terms of gross grasp and release. Surgical treatment and/or intramuscular neurolysis can sometimes result in both sensory and motor functional improvements, which for the hand are intimately related. Correction of the limb length difference is not expected.

In another case of hemiparesis post penetrating head injury with cerebritis, occupational therapy services were delayed 3 years, but significant hand function was regained once the services were instituted. Graphesthesia was not normal, but also was not absent in that patient.

In the present patient, brachial plexus palsy should have been notable at birth, since there is significant residual at this age. Brachial plexus palsy is associated with decreased reflexes and tone (though contracture could be confused with increased tone). In severe cases, the limb length difference is usually significantly greater than the relatively subtle difference seen in this patient.

Clinical Pearls

1. Pediatric disability can affect growth as well as function. Lower motor neuron lesions are affected more severely than upper.

2. Children who can't easily button their own shirts can wear t-shirts if their schools don't require a uniform. Families may suddenly notice deformities that have been present for a long time. This is also commonly the case in scoliosis: there may be an urgent concern about a chest deformity that in fact has slowly developed over time.

REFERENCES

1. Dahlin LB, Komoto-Tufvesson Y, Salgeback S: Surgery of the spastic hand in cerebral palsy. Improvement in stereognosis and hand function after surgery. J Hand Surg [Br] 23(3):334–339, 1998.
2. Eliasson AC, Ekholm C, Carlstedt T: Hand function in children with cerebral palsy after upper-limb tendon transfer and muscle release. Dev Med Child Neurol 40(9):612–621, 1998.
3. Gooch JL, Sandell TV: Botulinum toxin for spasticity and athetosis in children with cerebral palsy. Arch Phys Med Rehabil 77(5):508–511, 1996.
4. Van Heest AE, House J, Putnam M: Sensibility deficiencies in the hands of children with spastic hemiplegia. J Hand Surg [Am] 18(2):278–281, 1993.

PATIENT 42

A 41-year-old woman with progressive weakness

A 41-year-old woman presents with a slow-onset of upper and lower extremity weakness and sensory loss over the last several months. She has been healthy except for treatment for hypertension. She denies any history of trauma and gives no family history of health problems except for hypertension. She first noted the problem when she had more and more difficulty getting in and out of a chair and having more difficulty holding objects in her hands and writing. She denies any vision problems or swallowing problems. She comes to you for assessment and help with rehabilitation.

Physical Examination: Temperature 98.8°, pulse 85, respirations 16, blood pressure 140/78. HEENT: extra-occular movement intact, tongue in midline, facial movement symmetric. Chest: normal. Cardiac: normal. Abdomen: nontender, with normal active bowel sounds. Musculoskeletal: full range of motion of upper and lower extremities. Skin: normal. Neurologic: increased muscle tone in arms and legs; muscle stretch reflexes of upper and lower extremities 3/4; sustained ankle clonus bilaterally with a positive Babinski sign, bilaterally; 4/5 strength in left upper extremity and 3+/5 right upper extremity strength except for decreased grip strength of 2/5; 4/5 strength of the left lower extremity and 3+/5 strength of the right lower extremity; abnormal sensation to pinprick and light touch distal to C5 dermatome on right and C4 dermatome on left. Rectal: weak voluntary anal sphincter contraction; deep pressure sensation present, but abnormal sensation to pinprick or light touch.

Laboratory Findings: WBC 8700/μl; hct 38.5%; platelets 255,000/μl. BUN 6, creatinine 0.6 mg/dl, albumin g/dl. Urinalysis: normal. CSF: oligoclonal bands. Chest x-ray: no active pulmonary disease. CT scan of head: normal. MRI of head: normal. MRI of spine: see figure.

Question: What is the diagnosis?

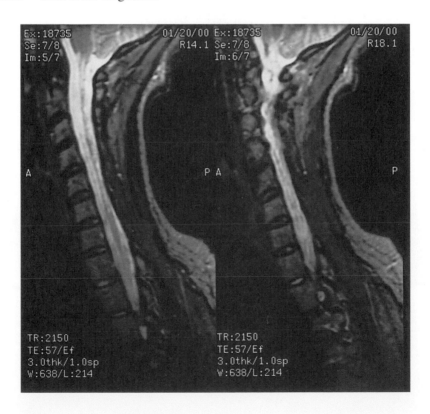

Diagnosis: Demyelinating plaque in the cervical spinal cord, probable multiple sclerosis.

Discussion: The diagnosis in this case is not straightforward. Multiple sclerosis is an inflammatory disease of unknown etiology of the central nervous system that is characterized by *mutiple* areas of **demyelination**. It is the third most common cause of disabling illness in persons aged 15–50 years. Individual symptoms are nonspecific, reflecting the *location* of the demyelinating lesions and not the disease process. Cerebrospinal fluid usually shows no specific abnormality. Protein is increased in 25% of patients during an exacerbation.

The oligoclonal nature of immunoglobulin G in the cerebrospinal fluid of individuals with multiple sclerosis has been demonstrated on agar gel electrophoresis. **Oligoclonal bands** in the cerebrospinal fluid are present in 90% of individuals with multiple sclerosis.

Magnetic resonance imaging is the preferred imaging tool to assist with the diagnosis. The demyelinating lesions are seen well with MRI—usually in the supratentorial white matter, especially in periventricular areas. The presence of three to four lesions > 3 mm in diameter is considered to be highly suspicious for multiple sclerosis.

The patient in this case had only a solitary lesion in the cervical spinal cord, which might be more characteristic of **transverse myelitis**. However, transverse myelitis is characterized by rapidly evolving paraparesis and not the slow onset that occurred in this patient. Tippet et al. found a series of patients with recurrent myelitis with only one locus of demyelination; despite great effort, no other lesions were detected on careful exam and MRI imaging. Some of the patients were noted to have oligoclonal bands in their cerebrospinal fluid. These bands sometimes occur with lupus erythematosus, mixed connective tissue disease, and antiphospholipid syndrome. The recurrent form is felt to be a type of multiple sclerosis.

In the present patient, surgical biopsy was performed to rule out tumor, as multiple sclerosis usually features multiple lesions. Biopsy revealed a large area of demyelination, but no inflammation. Her condition worsened clinically after surgery and she required ventilatory support; however, neurologic recovery was slow but sure. She was treated with steroids and intravenous immunoglobulin. After extensive 2-month inpatient rehabilitation, she was discharged to home walking with a rolling walker. Four months later at follow-up, she was able to ambulate short distances without any assistive devices. Unfortunately, she had another exacerbation 1 year later, experienced marked functional decline, and became wheelchair bound.

Clinical Pearls

1. Multiple sclerosis can present with a variety of symptoms, which are related to the *location* of the demyelinating plaque and not the disease process.

2. Multiple sclerosis is usually diagnosed with MRI evidence of multiple demyelinating plaques in the cerebrospinal fluid. A less recognized form has the appearance of transverse myelitis, except the latter does not feature slow onset and a recurrent disease pattern.

3. The presence of oligoclonal bands in the CSF is helpful but not diagnostic of multiple sclerosis.

REFERENCES

1. Adams RD, Victor M, Ropper AH: Multiple sclerosis and allied demyelinating diseases. In Principles of Neurology, 6th ed. New York, McGraw Hill, 1997.
2. Louenthal A, VanSande M, Koucher D: The differential diagnosis of neurological diseases by fractionating electrophoretically the CSF gamma globulins. J Neurochem 6:51–56, 1980.
3. Taylor RS: Rehabilitation of persons with multiple sclerosis. In Braddon RL (ed): Physical Medicine and Rehabilitation. Philadelphia, WB Saunders Co., 1996, pp 1101–1112.
4. Tippet DS, Fishman PS, Panitch HS: Recurrent transverse myelitis. Neurology 41:703, 1991.

PATIENT 43

A 50-year-old woman with low back pain radiating down both legs

A 50-year-old women is seeking medical treatment for an 11-month history of low back pain radiating down both legs. Her pain is worse on the right than on the left, and she has numbness in the right leg and foot. The pain began after she slid down the stairs at her home. While on a cruise, she noticed worsening with physical activity and radiating pain down her right leg and foot. She initially sought out chiropractic treatment. Radiographs obtained at that time did not reveal any evidence of lesions, fractures, dislocations, or significant degenerative changes. She then sought out the care of an orthopedic surgeon. Treatment was initiated with analgesics, muscle relaxants, anti-inflammatory drugs, and physical therapy. The treatment was unsuccessful, and the patient was referred for epidural steroid injections. Two epidural injections were slightly helpful in decreasing the right leg pain. However, she has not improved significantly.

The patient is a long-standing smoker and has lost 15 1bs in the last year. She underwent an excision of a large vaginal mass 4 years prior. Final histology at that time showed a smooth muscle tumor with no evidence of cellular atypia. Her most recent gynecological exam was unremarkable.

Physical Examination: Vital signs: normal. Neurologic: sensation diminished to light touch and pin prick in bilateral S1 distributions; all dermatomes and proprioception intact; reflexes absent at the ankles bilaterally, but other stretch reflexes intact and symmetric; radicular pain at 60° bilaterally on straight leg raising; 4/5 strength in ankle plantar flexors bilaterally, but otherwise normal results. Musculoskeletal: tenderness over right sacroiliac region and bilateral paraspinal musculature; trunk motion limited by pain in flexion.

Laboratory Findings: Lumbar lateral plain radiographs (see figure): decreased density in L3 vertebra, with scalloping and cortical erosion of inferior endplate; identified lumbosacral radiculopathy

Questions: What diagnostic imaging test and/or procedure would you obtain? What is the diagnosis?

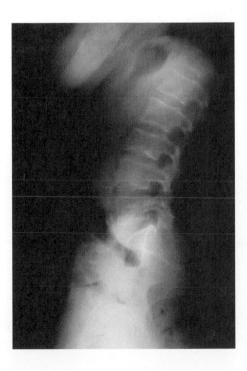

Answer: Lumbosacral MRI and open surgical biopsy. The diagnosis is metastatic uterine leiomyosarcoma, stage IV.

Discussion: **Uterine leiomyosarcoma** is one of the many types of uterine sarcomas. Sarcomas are malignancies arising from connective tissue. They rarely metastasize to the bone. Sarcomas have been classified into three categories: pure, mixed, and malignant mullerian tumors. Uterine leiomyosarcoma is a pure, homologous tumor of small smooth muscle arising from the myometrium. The cause is unknown; however, some sarcomas appear to be linked to prior radiotherapy. Peak incidence of leiomyosarcoma occurs in the 30- to 40-year age range and reaches a plateau in the middle-age period. It is most prevalent among African-American women and European American Jews. The diagnosis of leiomyosarcoma depends on histology. Atypia ranges from lesions that are well differentiated to anaplastic lesions that have the cytologic abnormalities of widely growing sarcomas.

The most common reported symptom in more than 80% of patients with a tumor involving the spine is back pain. Pain may be present even when recumbent. Radicular pain also may occur as a result of nerve root compression by an enlarging tumor or mass, or because of extrusion of boney fragments after a pathologic fracture. A neurologic deficit occurs in up to 70% of patients with spinal tumors, but is seldom present at initial presentation.

Weakness may not be manifested for months after onset of symptoms. Bowel and bladder symptoms may develop in as many as 50% of patients: they usually accompany lower extremity weakness and rarely occur as isolated symptoms.

Metastasis to the spine most commonly arises from carcinomas of the breast, lung, prostate, and, less frequently, from the kidney, thyroid gland, or gastrointestinal tract. The lumbar and thoracic spine is affected in approximately 45–49% of cases, with the cervical spine involved to a lesser degree. Most common causes of low back pain and radiculopathy are herniated nucleus pulposus and spinal stenosis. However, if the patient has persistent symptoms or is becoming worse despite appropriate treatment, then further investigation is warranted. Definitive diagnosis is imperative before performing invasive treatment to avoid delay in diagnosis of an infection or tumor.

Malignant tumors may be associated with rapid destruction of bone, including loss of posterior elements of the vertebral body. Plain radiographs do not demonstrate lesions until they are 1.0–1.5 cm in diameter or until 50–75% of the bone is destroyed. Plain radiographs are inexpensive and noninvasive, but they show lesions in only 60% of patients with metastatic bone disease. **Radionucleotide type scans** show metastasis in more than 95% of these patients. Radionucleotide type scans are highly sensitive, but nonspecific.

Magnetic resonance imaging is more sensitive than bone scintigraphy in detecting metastasis. Recent studies indicate an overall accuracy rate of 95%. MRI has an accuracy of 94% in differentiating benign from malignant spine fractures. Pathologic spine fractures typically have a low signal intensity on T1-weighted images and high signal intensity on T2-weighted images. These same changes may sometimes appear in benign lesions. To differentiate pathologic from benign lesions, the signal intensity and pattern of abnormal signal must be observed. Pathologic lesions display diffuse marrow infiltration of the pedicle and posterior element involvement. In addition gadolinum-diephylenetriamine pentaacetic acid (Gd-DTPA) as an intravenous paramagnetic contrast agent is especially useful in demonstrating epidural lesions and intradural extramedullary tumors.

In the present patient, a sagittal T1-weighted MRI (*left*) showed diffuse hypodensity in the L3 vertebra and a large presacral, intraspinal and soft tissue mass. A sagittal T2-weighted image (*right*) showed hyperdensity in the L3 vertebra and a large heterogeneous presacral, intraspinal, and soft tissue mass with regions of hyper- and hypointensity.

Approximately 50% of patients with **stage I** disease (confined to corpus uteri, 50% of all cases) survive longer than 5 years after diagnosis. **Stage II** disease is cancer involving the corpus and cervix, but not extending outside the uterus. **Stage III** disease is confined to the true pelvis. Patients with **stage IV** disease (cancer spreading to bowel, mucosa, or bladder, or metastasizing to different sites) have limited treatment options and are associated with a 5-year survival rate of 0–10%. Treatment for compressive lesions can be performed by surgical decompressive laminectomy. Chemotherapy can help in control of the metastatic spread of the disease.

Clinical Pearls

1. Low back and radicular pain may be secondary to metastatic and/or primary spine tumors.

2. Patients that have low back and/or radicular pain nonresponsive to conservative measures should receive appropriate diagnostic studies to exclude spinal malignancies.

3. MRI is more sensitive than bone scintigraphy in detecting metastasis to the spine.

4. Plain lumbosacral radiographs do not demonstrate lesions until they are 1.0–1.5 cm in diameter or until 50–75% of the bone is destroyed.

5. Uterine leiomyosarcoma can present as lumbosacral radiculopathy.

REFERENCES

1. Algra PR, Bloem JL, Tissing H, et al: Detection of Vertebral Metastases: Comparison between MR Imaging and Bone Scintigraphy. Radiographics 11; 129–132, 1991.
2. Botwin KB, Zak PJ: Lumbosacral radiculopathy secondary metastatic uterine leiomyosarcoma. A case report. Spine 25:884–887, 2000.
3. Copeland LJ: Uterine sarcomas. In: Textbook of Gynecology. Philadelphia, PA, WB Saunders, 1993, pp 1034–1041.
4. Hart RA, Weinstein J: Primary and Benign and Malignant Musculoskeletal Tumors of the Spine. Semin Spine Surg 7: 288–302, 1995.
5. Li KC, Poon FY: Sensitivity and Specificity of MRI in Detecting Malignant Spinal Cord Compression and Distinguishing Malignant from Benign Compression Fractures of Vertebrae. Magn Reson Imaging 6: 547-556, 1998.
6. Salazar H: Uterine Sarcomas: Natural History, Treatment and Prognosis. Cancer 42:1152,1978.

PATIENT 44

A 36-year-old woman with shoulder pain

A 36-year-old, right-handed woman presents with right shoulder pain. Onset was gradual, beginning 2 months ago. There is no injury involved. She describes the pain as an ache, and she has some limitation of movement, but no swelling. The patient is able to perform most of her usual activities. There is no neck pain or radicular symptoms. She has no fever, chills, or neurologic symptoms. Past history is significant for bilateral hip pain.

Physical Examination: Musculoskeletal: mild tenderness of right shoulder, no erythema or warmth; range of motion (ROM) somewhat restricted, more so on internal and external rotation than on flexion-abduction arc; rotator cuff impingement signs absent. Cervical spine: normal. Neurologic: normal.

Laboratory Findings: X-ray of shoulder (see below): partial density of humeral head.

Questions: Which disorders and activities should this patient be questioned about? What is the diagnosis?

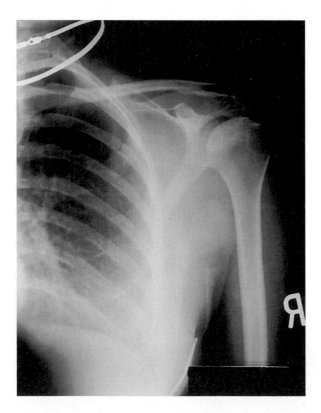

Answers: Query the patient about a history of systemic disorder such as systemic lupus erythematosus (SLE) or rheumatoid arthritis, long-term steroid use, alcoholism, blood and coagulation disorders, lymphoma or cancer, metabolic diseases, and deep sea diving. The diagnosis is avascular necrosis of the right shoulder and bilateral hips (multifocal osteonecrosis).

Discussion: Multifocal osteonecrosis is defined as disease involving three or more anatomic sites. It affects the humeral and femoral heads most often, and in the majority of cases is associated with conditions like alcohol abuse or steroid therapy.

Most patients with shoulder pain due to nontraumatic osteonecrosis have a lesion involving the head of the humerus, on one or both sides. The lesion usually starts as an osteolytic area in the subchondral bone and progresses to collapse. Articular cartilage separates from subchondral bone and either becomes a detached free cap or reattaches at a later stage. Patients in whom the condition develops can have: (1) a minimal lesion that heals well, (2) a moderate deformity that is well tolerated, or (3) severe joint disease requiring surgical correction.

Nontraumatic osteonecrosis results from circulatory impairment to the affected bone. The femoral head is affected most often. Steroid use, alcohol consumption, pancreatitis, and lipid disorders appear to lead to bone death either by development of fat emboli in the microcirculature surrounding the affected bone or by fatty infiltration of the marrow. Decompression syndrome results from the presence of gaseous emboli in the microcirculature. Other frequently suggested pathogenic factors that play a role in the development of osteonecrosis include increased intraosseous pressures, the presence of cytotoxic cellular factors, intravascular coagulation, venous stasis, and the hyperviscosity syndrome. In addition, patients have developed osteonecrosis without any known risk factors; this syndrome has been coined idiopathic avascular necrosis.

In patients with a diagnosis of osteonecrosis and complaints in other joints, these other areas should be fully evaluated with plain radiographs and, if inconclusive, with bone scan or MRI. In patients with osteonecrosis not involving the femoral head, the patient's hips should be radiographically evaluated regardless of whether the patient is symptomatic. Evaluate other joints in patients diagnosed with osteonecrosis of the knee, shoulder, or ankle, as such patients have multifocal disease roughly 50% of the time.

In a large study, 151 patients with 200 shoulders affected with osteonecrosis of the humeral head were evaluated for associated factors, the need for prosthetic replacement surgery, the state of the unoperated shoulder, and the existence of prognostic factors. Associated factors included corticosteroid use in 112 shoulders, trauma in 37, Gaucher's disease in 3, sickle cell disease in 3, and radiation necrosis in 1. No cause was evident in 44 shoulders. Ninety-seven shoulders required replacement surgery.

Early diagnosis of this condition is essential especially in the weight-bearing joints to avoid the need for replacement surgery. Bone scan or MRI are common measures for diagnosis if x-rays are normal. MRI can detect early changes of osteonecrosis, such as poorly defined marrow edema. Proper staging of the disease is also important after a correct diagnosis is made. Treatment is nonsurgical for early stages in the non-weight bearing joints. Minimally invasive outpatient surgery such as core-decompression or drilling holes in the subchondral bone to improve vascular supply is not as widely popular in shoulders compared to hips; however, recent studies have shown good outcomes even for advanced stages II and III osteonecrosis in terms of early relief of pain and increased function. Less than 50% patients with affected shoulders require replacement surgery.

In the present patient, further questioning revealed the presence of SLE, as well as chronic steroid use for the disorder. X-rays showed various stages of osteonecrosis. The far-advanced disease in her hips was not suitable for core decompression. She underwent left hip replacement (see figure below), with the understanding that the opposite hip would soon need replacing. Core decompression of her shoulder reduced the pain and improved range of movement and function.

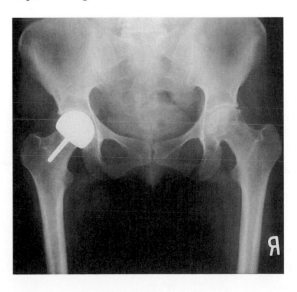

Clinical Pearls

1. Multifocal osteonecrosis involves three or more anatomic sites. Most common sites are the femur and humerus heads.

2. Lesions usually start as an osteolytic area in the subchondral bone and progress to collapse.

3. Microcirculatory impairment, increased intraosseous pressures, the presence of cytotoxic cellular factors, intravascular coagulation, venous stasis, and hyperviscosity are the most important pathogenic factors.

4. Aggressively investigate painful joints for the presence of osteonecrosis in patients with chronic steroid use. Bone scan is a very sensitive modality, but MRI is more specific and at least as sensitive.

5. Core decompression of the shoulder is a safe procedure with few recognized complications and can be performed on an outpatient basis. The procedure has been successful for Stages I, II, and III osteonecrosis in terms of early relief of pain and increased function.

REFERENCES

1. Collaborative Osteonecrosis Group: Symptomatic multifocal osteonecrosis. A multicenter study. 369:312–326, 1999.
3. Hattrup SJ, Cofield RH: Osteonecrosis of the humeral head: Relationship of disease stage, extent, and cause to natural history. J Shoulder Elbow Surg 8:559–564, 1999.
2. Cruess RL: Corticosteroid-induced osteonecrosis of the humeral head. Orthop Clin North Am 16:789–796, 1985.
4. LaPorte DM, Mont MA, Mohan V, et al : Multifocal osteonecrosis. 25:1968–1974, 1998.

PATIENT 45

A 34-year-old man with a history of left below-elbow amputation

A 34-year-old man complains of a 6-month history of perceived pain in his amputated hand. He was employed as a tree surgeon until 1 year ago, when he was involved in an accident resulting in a violent amputation of his left forearm by a dropped chainsaw. He reports that he had no hand pain prior to the amputation. The quality of the pain is described as burning with some pins-and-needles sensation. The pain is intermittent, but seems to interfere with daily functions. The patient currently uses a body-powered prosthesis with a figure-eight harness, locking wrist unit, and #7 heavy-duty terminal device. The patient's socket is a double-wall plastic laminate with a Bowen single control cable used to activate the terminal device. He is presently taking a combination of gabapentin and trazodone for pain relief and insomnia. The patient reports no history of neuroma or excessive pain at the end of his stump. He is currently unemployed and is receiving partial Social Security Disability.

Physical Examination: General: well developed, no distress. Temperatures: residual limb 28° C; right limb 31° C. Musculoskeletal: residual stump length 10 cm distal to lateral epicondyle; full active and passive range of motion in shoulder and elbow. Neurologic: sensation intact to pinprick and two-point discrimination in residual stump.

Laboratory Findings: CBC, electrolytes, ESR: normal.

Question: What type of pain is this patient experiencing?

Answer: Phantom limb pain.

Discussion: Phantom limb pain is described as pain that affects the parts of the limb that have been lost due to traumatic amputation or another form of denervation, such as seen in paraplegia. Attempts have been made to differentiate forms of sensory input of the phantom limb. "Pain in the residual limb" refers to pain in the stump of an extremity amputation. "Phantom sensation" describes any sensation—except pain—in the absent limb. Many studies have failed to distinguish these phenomena; therefore, consensus on the etiology of phantom limb pain is controversial. This discussion attempts to outline some of the more common theories.

The prevalence of phantom limb pain is also a controversial topic. Many studies suggest that phantom limb pain is rare; however, others report that 60–85% of amputees experience some form of phantom limb pain. The intensity of these pain phenomena has been reported to be similar to that of chronic low back pain, cancer pain, and labor pain. Phantom pain is usually located or perceived in the distal part of the amputated limb. The quality of the pain is often variable, but most commonly referred to as "burning" or "cramping."

Treatments have been categorized according to the type of pain reported by the patient. Unfortunately, all treatments to this point have had less than favorable responses. Patients commonly describe the pain as similar to pre-amputation pain. This description is especially typical in older patients who have a variety of comorbidities, including peripheral neuropathy and peripheral vascular disease. Some research shows the incidence of phantom limb pain to be greater in male populations; other studies show no difference between genders. There does appear to be a consistent relationship between temperature and phantom limb pain. When patients report throbbing or burning pain, the temperature of the stump tends to be significantly lower than in the intact opposite limb.

The explanations for the pathophysiology of phantom limb pain are varied. Early theories tended to center on **peripherally based etiologies**. It was believed that neuromas resulting from the ends of cut nerves generated impulses to the central nervous system, which resulted in the perception of phantom limb pain. This hypothesis has been supported by the fact that phantom limb pain is more frequent in patients with pathology involving the stump, such as neuromas, fissures, and excessive scar tissue. Peripheral pathology definitely plays some role in phantom limb pain, but cannot be the sole etiology because the pain has been reported immediately after amputation. Additionally, there are many patients with significant stump pathology who have no phantom pain whatsoever.

Other theories for the development of phantom limb pain center on the **brain and spinal cord**. Phantom limb pain may be due to abnormal firing patterns in internuncial neurons in the spinal cord or to alterations in higher brain centers. Brain alterations described as input-decreased cortical reorganization in the somatosensory cortex, with immunocytochemical evidence of hyperexcitability in the thalamus, have been shown in patients with phantom limb pain. The reticular activating system may play an important role, as well: a disinhibition occurs, resulting in synchronous, self-sustaining activity that can be perceived as pain.

Yet another explanation for phantom limb pain includes **psychological disorders**. Patients with personality features such as compulsive self-reliance and rigidity report higher incidence of phantom limb pain. Other psychological explanations associate defense mechanisms such as denial or repression with higher incidents of phantom limb pain. Depression can be an important part of the overall concept of phantom limb pain; amputation can profoundly effect the psychological health of an individual.

One theory that has attempted to combine the multifaceted nature of phantom limb pain—the **neuromatrix theory**, described by Melzack—involves three major circuits in the brain that connect the somatosensory cortex, the reticular formation leading to the limbic system, and the parietal lobe. The concept is that pain comes into our conscious awareness by the processing of information in these highly connected circuits. The connections themselves also are able to produce some sensory information. This theory implies that many facets of an amputee's experience, including peripheral sensory input, the neuromatrix, and psychological and social factors, lead to the experience of phantom limb pain.

A combination of these theories is likely, as treatment of each etiology as a separate entity has not proven to be effective. Treatments for phantom limb pain are varied. They include pharmacotherapy, peripheral nerve blocks, sympathetic blocks, and nerve stimulation. A recent study describes the use of a Sauerbruch prosthesis resulting in decreased phantom limb pain perception, compared to a control group that used a cosmetic prosthesis. The presumed mechanism for this improvement would be an increase in use-dependent cortical reorganization of the afferent-decrease type that highly correlates with phantom limb pain. However, this study was small, and it should be repeated with higher numbers of patients for validity.

Clinical Pearls

1. Phantom limb pain refers to pain perceived to be in a portion of an amputated limb. This is to be distinguished from pain in the stump.

2. The pathophysiology of phantom limb pain is controversial, but seems to involve multiple sources, including input from peripheral, spinal, and cortical centers.

3. Treatment of phantom limb pain includes pharmacotherapy, peripheral and sympathetic nerve blocks, and screening for mood disorders.

REFERENCES

1. Hill A: Phantom limb pain: A review of the literature on attributes and potential mechanisms. 17(2):125–139,1999.
2. Weiss T, Miltner W, Adler T, et al: Decrease in phantom limb pain associated with prosthesis-induced increased use of an amputated stump in humans. Neurosci Lett 272:131–134, 1999.

PATIENT 46

A 64-year-old man with cough and shortness of breath

A 64-year-old man presents with a 3-month history of cough and shortness of breath. He experiences these symptoms primarily while eating. The patient's wife and friends began to notice that he was slurring his speech. This problem did not improve over the course of several weeks. He refused to see a doctor, but changed his mind when painful cramps developed in his lower extremities. He denies fever, chills, visual changes, and bowel/bladder incontinence, and has not noticed generalized fatigue. He has a medical history of hypertension, hiatal hernia, and peripheral vascular disease. He has smoked three cigars per day for the past 10 years.

Physical Examination: Temperature 98.9°, pulse 84 and regular, blood pressure 145/88, respirations 22. Oral cavity: increased saliva, no sputum or erythema. Neck: no nuchal rigidity, good range of motion, 1+ carotid pulses, normal nodes. Cardiac: regular rate and rhythm, with no murmurs. Chest: clear except for transmitted sounds from upper airways. Abdomen: nontender, normal sounds. Extremities: no clubbing, cyanosis, or edema. Neurologic: reduced gag reflex and mild weakness in sternocleidomastoids; remaining cranial nerves normal; normal sensory; 4+/5 strength in proximal muscles of upper and lower limbs; brisk reflexes in all extremities.

Question: What diagnostic test would be most helpful in arriving at a diagnosis?

Answer: Electromyography/nerve conduction study

Discussion: A nerve conduction study of the present patient revealed normal motor and sensory nerve activity. Electromyography (EMG) revealed fibrillations and positive sharp waves in the distal muscles of all four extremities, in addition to fasciculation potentials in three distal extremities along with the genioglossus muscle. Motor units had large amplitudes and reduced recruitment pattern. The diagnosis is amyotrophic lateral sclerosis (ALS).

ALS is a progressive, degenerative, neurologic disorder in which motor units in the central nervous system are lost. The incidence is 1–3 per 100,000 population; the male to female ratio is 2 to 1. ALS usually presents in the seventh decade. Both upper and lower motor neuron signs and symptoms involving bulbar, respiratory, and limb muscles are present. The clinical course involves progressive weakness, cramping, **fasciculations**, atrophy, spasticity, and **respiratory decline**. Bulbar signs such as dysphagia and dysarthria usually present early in the disease course. Eventually, as respiratory and bulbar motor function deteriorate more, respiratory failure results in ventilator dependence and, eventually, death.

Although the etiology of ALS is not known, recent studies suggest that a genetic mutation in the gene that codes for Cu/Zn superoxide dismutase 1 on chromosome 21 may be a factor. Other possible etiologies include autoimmunity, free radical toxicity, and over-active glutamate receptors. ALS spares bowel and bladder function and tends to spare sensory and oculomotor function.

One in four people present with bulbar paralysis; these individuals have the poorest prognosis. Bulbar signs tend to present earlier in older individuals. People with disease onset at an earlier age have a much longer survival time. Although ALS is considered to feature an accelerated course toward death, up to 22% of patients survive more than 10 years without ventilatory support.

The presentation and clinical course of ALS can be quite variable. As illustrated in the present patient with dysphagia, bulbar signs may present prior to limb or trunk signs. The weakness may present proximally before distally; however, distal weakness usually occurs first. While **classic ALS** involves upper and lower motor neurons of bulbar, trunk, and limb muscles, three other types of ALS also are described:

• **Progressive bulbar palsy**—a strictly bulbar form
• **Primary lateral sclerosis**—a strictly upper motor neuron type
• **Progressive muscular atrophy**—an entirely lower motor neuron form.

The classic presentation is seen 90% of the time, and there is much debate regarding whether the other three classifications really exist as separate entities.

Disagreement exists regarding the proper use of exercise in ALS patients, but there is general agreement that strengthening exercises are effective for the less weakened muscles in patients with a slower disease course. The present patient, due to his very rapid course, received physical therapy/occupational therapy concentrating on stretching, passive range of motion, and energy conservation. He required a gastrostomy tube 6 months after his confirmed diagnosis. An augmentative communication device was required around the time of the feeding tube placement. He started using an electric wheelchair 1 month later, and a portable ventilator soon after that. His family, friends, and rehabilitation staff were very supportive during his disease progression. The patient died of aspiration pneumonia 18 months after the onset of his disease.

Clinical Pearls

1. The etiology of ALS is unknown, but possible causes include a genetic mutation of a gene coding for superoxide dismutase, autoimmunity, free radical toxicity, or over-active glutamate receptors.

2. Of patients with ALS, 25% present with bulbar paralysis. These individuals tend to be older, and they have the poorest prognosis.

3. Up to 22% of people with ALS survive more than 10 years without ventilatory support.

4. The appropriate use of exercise in patients with ALS is debatable. However, physicians generally agree that strengthening exercises are effective for less weakened muscles in those with a slower disease course.

5. *Classic* ALS accounts for 90% of the cases, and involves upper and lower motor neurons of bulbar, trunk, and limb muscles. There is controversy as to whether the three other forms of ALS actually exist as separate entities.

REFERENCES

1. Agre JC, Matthews DJ: Rehabilitation concepts in motor neuron diseases. In Braddom RL (ed): Physical Medicine and Rehabilitation. Philadelphia, WB Saunders Company, 1996, pp 955–971.
2. Francis K, Bach JR, DeLisa JA: Evaluation and rehabilitation of patients with adult motor neuron disease. Arch Phys Med Rehabil 80:951–963, 1999.
3. Kirsteins AE, Kolaski K: Neuromuscular diseases. In Grabois M, Garrison SJ, Hart KA, Lehmkuhl LD (eds): Physical Medicine and Rehabilitation: The Complete Approach. Malden, MA, Blackwell Science, 2000, pp 1649–1652.
4. Wilbourn AJ: Electrodiagnostic evaluation of the suspected ALS patient. In Belsh JM, Schiffman PL (eds): Amyotrophic Lateral Sclerosis: Diagnosis and Management for the Clinician. Armonk, New York, Futura Publishing Co., Inc, 1996, pp 163–202.

PATIENT 47

A 72-year-old man with a traumatic brain injury
and difficulty swallowing

A 72-year-old man was injured in a fall from a ladder and suffered a moderate traumatic brain injury requiring inpatient rehabilitation care for about a month. Prior to his injury he was independent in all activities of daily living, including driving, balancing a checkbook, and reading at college level. During the course of his recovery, his speech and language skills improved to near baseline level; motor function recovered to nearly the same extent; and short- and long-term memory recovered to his pre-morbid status. However, a nasogastric feeding tube is still being used for thin liquids nearly 4 weeks after admission to the traumatic brain injury rehabilitation unit, because a videofluoroscopic swallowing study repeatedly demonstrated "silent" aspiration of thin liquids. In all other areas of motor, cognitive, and psychological function, the patient has nearly complete recovery.

Physical Examination: General: thin; no acute distress. Neurologic: cranial nerve I not tested; II—visual acuity normal; III, IV, and VI—extraocular muscles intact; V—mastication muscles normal; VII—face symmetric; VIII—hearing normal; IX and X—abnormal soft palate elevation with phonation, gag reflex diminished; XI—shrug symmetric; XII—tongue midline in position, hyperactive jaw jerk.

Laboratory Findings: CT scan of head: resolving hemorrhages in prefrontal cortex. Serum electrolytes, blood counts, and cerebrospinal fluids: normal. EMG: occasional fasciculations in sample muscles tested in three of four limbs; also in tongue.

Question: What is the diagnosis?

Diagnosis: Amyotrophic lateral sclerosis

Discussion: Although a traumatic brain injury could account for this patient's difficulty in swallowing, it is unlikely that this profound problem would persist while such extensive neurologic recovery was made in other areas (motor, cognitive, memory, and speech). The key to the answer is found in the physical exam and EMG test. Note that the soft palate did not normally elevate with phonation, which accounts for the dysphagia. But also notice that there was a hyperactive jaw jerk. These symptoms—**weakness of the soft palate, hyporeflexia of the gag reflex, and a hyperactive jaw jerk reflex**—provide evidence for both lower motor neuron (weakness and hyporeflexia) and upper motor neuron (hyperactive reflexes) involvement. Moreover, the EMG exam further demonstrates lower motor neuron abnormalities: fasciculations. Taken together, these findings are not consistent with a traumatic brain injury, which is an upper motor neuron problem, but rather with a disorder affecting both upper and lower motor neurons: amyotrophic lateral sclerosis (ALS).

ALS, also known as Lou Gehrig's disease, is one of the most common progressive neuromuscular diseases, affecting 5 to 7 individuals per 100,000. ALS is a motor neuron disease that results in destruction of both upper and lower motor neurons. It most commonly affects individuals aged 40 to 60 years, with a mean age of onset of 58. Men are more commonly affected than women by a 3:2 ratio. Poor prognostic signs include old age at onset, bulbar findings, fasciculations in all limbs, and time from onset of symptoms to diagnosis.

ALS commonly presents with both upper and lower motor neuron findings. Thus, the clinician should suspect a diagnosis of ALS in any elderly male with both lower motor neuron abnormalities (weakness, hyporeflexia, fasciculations), and upper motor neuron abnormalities (spasticity, hyperactive reflexes, Hoffman's sign).

Physical therapy in patients with ALS is directed toward optimizing physical function while planning for future quality of life. Stretching exercises may help prevent joint immobility, and aerobic exercise can improve cardiovascular function and minimize fatigue, but patients should not exercise to the point of muscle overuse. Signs of overwork include delayed-onset muscle soreness, post-exercise weakness, and muscle cramping.

Dysarthria and dysphagia often result due to both upper and lower motor neuron loss in ALS patients. In contrast, traumatic brain injuries result in dysarthria and dysphagia only in severe cases, and are generally associated with other clinical findings, such as spasticity of the limbs, cognitive dysfunction, and trouble with balance and coordination. The present patient made good neurologic recovery in these areas, yet still experienced profound difficulty in swallowing that seemed out of concordance with his overall recovery. Accordingly, attention was focused on the existence of another concurrent disease entity to explain these unexpected findings. The EMG exam uncovered additional lower motor neuron abnormalities that confirmed the diagnosis of ALS.

Clinical Pearls

1. In ALS patients, the presence of fasciculations in multiple limbs on EMG exam is associated with a poor prognosis.
2. A diagnosis of ALS should be considered in any elderly individual with fasciculations and swallowing difficulty.

REFERENCES

1. Hillel AD, Miller R: Bulbar amyotrophic lateral sclerosis: Patterns of progression and clinical management [see comments]. Head Neck 11:51–59, 1989.
2. Jackson CE, Bryan WW: Amyotrophic lateral sclerosis. Semin Neurol 18:27–39, 1998.
3. Sliwa JA: Neuromuscular rehabilitation and electrodiagnosis. 1. Central neurologic disorders. Arch Phys Med Rehabil 81:S3–12, 2000.
4. Walling AD: Amyotrophic lateral sclerosis: Lou Gehrig's disease [see comments]. Am Fam Physician 59:1489–1496, 1999.

PATIENT 48

A 28-year-old man with left foot drop post surgery

A 28-year-old man is referred from Neurosurgery for evaluation of his left foot drop. By history, the foot drop began after a lumbar laminectomy to correct an L4-L5 herniated nucleus propulsus. He denies any difficulty with his gait prior to that time, except for "difficulty with walking" following an injury sustained in a parachute jump while in the army 2 years prior to his surgery. His ability to walk easily improved with time. An electrodiagnostic test is now requested to rule out an acute nerve injury secondary to the surgery.

Physical Examination: General: well-developed and muscular. Gait: reciprocal, with left foot drop and compensatory left hip hike. Musculoskeletal: right lower extremity 5/5 strength, left lower extremity 5/5 strength except for dorsiflexion, great toe extension, eversion 1/5 strength. Neurologic: sensation impaired to light touch in left L5 dermatome; reflexes normal and symmetric, except for absent left hamstring reflex.

Laboratory Findings: See results of nerve conduction and EMG studies below.

Question: Do the study results rule out an acute nerve injury?

Nerve Conduction Study

Nerve	Site	Latency	CV	Amplitude
L deep peroneal	Ankle-EDB	4.3 msec		6.0 mV
	FH-ankle		46 m/s	5.2 mV
	Pop fossa-FH		44 m/s	4.9 mV
L sural (sensory)	Mid-calf-ankle	3.7 msec	37.8 m/s	18 µV
R deep peroneal	Ankle-EDB	4.5 msec		10 mV
	FH-ankle		48 m/s	9.6 mV
	Pop fossa-FH		50 m/s	9.3 mV
R sural (sensory)	Mid-calf-ankle	3.6 msec	38.9 m/s	25 µV
L tibial H-reflex		38.5 msec		
R tibial H-reflex		39.1 msec		

CV = conduction velocity, EDB = extensor digitorum brevis, FH = fibular head, m/s = meters/second

EMG Study

Muscle	Insertional Activity	MUAP morphology	MUAP recruitment
L L2-5 paraspinals	Normal	—	—
L vastus medialis	Normal	Normal	Normal
L anterior tibialis	Normal	Large amplitude	Few MUAP seen
L peroneus longus	Normal	Large amplitude	Decreased
L medial gastroc	Normal	Normal	Normal
L short head-biceps	Normal	Normal	Normal
L gluteus medius	Normal	Large amplitude	Mildly decreased

MUAP = motor unit action potential

Diagnosis: Old L5 radiculopathy with evidence of reinnervation but no evidence of acute denervation

Discussion: Time-related events are important sign-posts for the diagnostician. As in this case, the exact time of injury could not be determined by history. If the nerve injury, as reported by this patient, had occurred 2 months prior to the testing, the presence of spontaneous activity such as fibrillation and positive sharp wave potentials in the paraspinal and limb muscles would be expected. After 2 months post-injury, the motor unit action potential (MUAP) morphology should demonstrate more polyphasic waveforms due to collateral sprouting. Insufficient time had elapsed for development of large amplitude MUAP as was present on this patient's needle examination. With significant axonal loss, there would be MUAP "dropout," corresponding with decreased recruitment and interference patterns.

Following axonal nerve injury, diverse events occur patho-physiologically. Some of these events can be detected by electrodiagnostic studies. These events may assist the diagnostician in determining the age of the injury. During the first day after partial or complete nerve transection, the distal stump begins swelling. Within the first several days there is axoplasmic disruption, fragmentation of the neural tubules and neurofilaments, and fragmentation between the nodes of Ranvier. By the fifth day, further degradation is produced by a proliferation of Schwann cells and macrophages. This degradation continues over the next several weeks. Initially, the neuromuscular junction and slow-axonal transport system continue to function. On the EMG needle exam, there should be no signs of muscle membrane instability, such as fibrillation potentials and positive sharp waves. If any voluntary muscle activity is present, the morphology of the MUAP should be normal, with decreased recruitment and interference patterns. Compound motor action potentials (CMAPs) and sensory nerve action potentials (SNAPs) amplitudes and latencies will be normal distal to the site of injury.

Wallerian degeneration begins at about the fifth day. On EMG study, spontaneous activity may be seen in muscles that are in close proximity to the injury (such as paraspinal muscles in the case of radiculopathy), but still is not present in the more distal musculature. The neuromuscular junction fails about 5 days after a complete nerve transection and, therefore, a CMAP cannot be obtained after that. End-plate potentials also disappear. Muscle fiber atrophy begins within 1 week. The muscle fibers have a reduction in their resting membrane

potential. An increased sensitivity of extrajunctional muscle membrane to acetylcholine contributes to fibrillation potentials. With partial nerve transection, CMAPs and SNAPs have reduced amplitudes; nerve conduction velocities and latencies may or may not be affected depending on whether or not the fastest conducting fibers were severed.

At 2–3 weeks, depolarization continues due to reduction in the electrogenic activity of the sodium pumping mechanism of the muscle membrane. Resting muscle membrane permeability decreases to potassium and increases to sodium. Acetylcholine receptors begin appearing outside the synaptic region. Fibrillation and positive sharp wave potentials begin to appear in the distal musculature. In general, the amount of fibrillation potentials and positive sharp waves that are present correspond to the extent of the nerve damage.

Within the first day following injury, the proximal nerve stump begins to sprout. The sprouts usually are seen distal to the injury site within 4 to 10 days. Depending on the damage to the distal portion of the endoneurial tube, the sprouts grow at a rate of 1–4 millimeters per day. With partial nerve injury, reinnervation of the orphan muscle fibers begins by sprouting of the undamaged axons that are within close proximity. Regeneration of the injured axon occurs at about 2–3 millimeters per day. On EMG, polyphasic MUAPs are evidence of the sprouting. The polyphasic MUAPs are due to the immature myelin on the sprouts, leading to desynchronization of the MUAPs. The area under the polyphasic MUAP curve should correspond to the number of muscle fibers innervated by that axon. The regenerating axons begin to mature once they reach their destination.

As the myelin of the nerve sprouts mature, the MUAPs become more synchronized, which causes larger amplitudes. This synchronization occurs at about 6 months post injury. With reinnervation, the spontaneous activity may continue, but should be smaller in amplitude and amount than spontaneous activity found on earlier needle examination.

In the present patient, the electrodiagnostic testing did not reveal any spontaneous activity or polyphasic MUAPs in any of the muscles tested. The spontaneous activity or morphologic changes of the MUAPs would have supported the patient's claim that his injury was due to the surgery. Instead, the MUAPs that were evaluated had large amplitudes, a finding that supports his injury being at least 6 months old.

Clinical Pearls

1. Presence of polyphasic or giant amplitude MUAPs helps determine the time since a nerve injury.

2. Amplitudes of spontaneous activity in the muscle should decrease with time.

3. For radiculopathies, denervation or reinnervation changes should be restricted to single root level, with abnormalities confirmed in at lease two limb muscles innervated by different peripheral branches of that same root.

REFERENCES

1. Dumitru D. Reaction of the peripheral nervous system to injury. In Dumitru D (ed): Electrodiagnostic Medicine. Philadelphia, Hanley & Belfus, Inc., 1995, pp 341–384.
2. Dorfman LJ: Quantitative clinical electrophysiology in the evaluation of nerve injury and regeneration. Muscle Nerve 13:822–828, 1990.
3. Kraft GH: Fibrillation potential amplitude and muscle atrophy following peripheral nerve injury. Muscle Nerve 13:814–821, 1990.
4. Robinson LR: Traumatic injury to peripheral nerves. Muscle Nerve 23:63–73, 2000.

PATIENT 49

A 75-year-old man with stroke, left hemiparesis, and left lower extremity pain

A 75-year-old man sustained left hemiparesis 5 months ago from a right thalamic stroke. He underwent rehabilitation and achieved modified independence in ambulation by using a straight cane. However, severe, burning, and deep left-sided pain has gradually developed. He also complains of extreme sensitivity of his left upper and lower extremities to any type of stimulation, and the touch of a breeze or light blanket worsens his symptoms.

Physical Examination: Blood pressure 135/75, pulse 90, respiration 20, temperature 97.9°. Neurologic: alert and oriented to person, place, time, and self; mild distress due to pain; light touch to left lower limb elicited complaints of pain. Musculoskeletal: 3/5–4/5 in left upper and lower extremities, 5/5 in right upper and lower extremities; muscle tone mildly increased; muscle stretch reflexes increased (+3) on left; left lower extremity very tender to light palpation. Skin: no warmth or redness.

Laboratory Findings: WBC 7200/μl, Hct 45%, platelets 298,00/μl. ESR 7 mm/hr. D-dimer assay: negative. Left lower extremity venous Doppler: negative for deep venous thrombosis. X-rays of femur and tibia-fibula: negative for fracture or dislocation. Triple-phase bone scan: normal.

Question: What is the cause of this patient's pain?

Diagnosis: Central post-stroke pain

Discussion: Central post-stroke pain, also known as thalamic pain or Dejerine-Roussy syndrome, has a low incidence and occurs in 1.5–5% of patients who survive a stroke episode. Pain sensations vary from dull and achy to sharp and shooting; pain is typically diffuse, intense, and severe. Physical examination findings are minimal to none. **Allodynia**, which is the perception of pain to a benign stimulus, is often elicited.

Patients with central post-stroke pain usually have thalamic infarcts or hemorrhages, but some may have cerebrovascular lesions in other areas of the brain. The actual mechanism is unknown. But there is evidence from studies with somatosensory evoked potentials that there are somatosensory tract abnormalities, indicating a release phenomenon.

The diagnosis is based on exclusion. It is important to identify other causes of pain, such as a deep venous thrombosis, fracture or dislocation, and complex regional pain syndromes (CRPS) types I and II. In the present patient, all studies pertaining to these diagnoses were negative. In addition, CRPS type I (also known as reflex sympathetic dystrophy) presents with more focal pain related to an extremity and/or joint. CRPS type II, or causalgia, presents with pain limited to a peripheral nerve distribution.

Treatment of central post-stroke pain is difficult. It requires comprehensive management and includes supportive measures (prevention of skin problems, avoidance of noxious stimuli, good overall hygiene), range-of motion exercises, and maximizing use of the weaker side. Medications are often prescribed, and they range from simple analgesics to anticonvulsants and antidepressants. Psychotherapy, relaxation training, and hypnosis are also employed.

The present patient experienced partial relief with a combination of an anticonvulsant drug and psychotherapy.

Clinical Pearls

1. The incidence of central post-stroke pain is low (1.5–5%), but it is an important entity that can produce disabling pain.

2. Patients with central post-stroke pain may have cerebrovascular lesions in areas other than the thalamus.

3. Central post-stroke pain presents in a diffuse pattern, in comparison to complex regional pain syndromes types I and II, which present with more localized pain.

REFERENCES
1. Kirsteins AE, Black-Schaffer RM, Harvey RL: Stroke rehabilitation. 3. Rehabilitation management. Arch Phys Med Rehabil 80:S17–S20, 1999.
2. Roth EJ: Medical complications encountered in stroke rehabilitation. PM&R Clin North Am 2(3):563–578, 1991.
3. Roth EJ: Stroke. In O'Young B, Young MA, Stiens SA (eds): PM&R Secrets. Philadelphia, Hanley & Belfus, 1997.

PATIENT 50

A 17-year-old girl with cerebral palsy and new-onset edema

A 17-year-old girl with moderate to severe spastic diplegic cerebral palsy presents with increasing swelling of both legs over the last several months. The swelling is now interfering with her orthotic use. Her physical therapist is alarmed because the patient has lost her limited walking ability (about 100 feet, using ankle-foot orthotics and a walker, and with supervision) and is having difficulty with transfers and activities of daily living. Multiple releases were performed at age 4, and since then she has been on baclofen intermittently; due to her current difficulties, she has resumed taking 10 mg BID. She has some hip pain attributed to subchondral sclerosis, noted on a pelvis x-ray at age 16, and also takes ibuprofen 400 mg TID. There is no dysphagia, nor bladder or bowel incontinence. A study for carpal tunnel syndrome a year ago, due to complaints of wrist pain, was negative. A Doppler venous examination of the lower extremities done when the swelling was milder was negative. Compressive stockings were prescribed.

Physical Examination: General: weight 82.5 kg, height estimated 4' 8" (weight 58.4 kg 18 months ago). HEENT: unremarkable. Cardiac: regular rate and rhythm, no abnormal sound. Chest: clear. Abdomen: palpation difficult due to obesity, but benign; no obvious masses or organomegaly. Extremities: significant swelling of all four limbs, more in the legs, and non-pitting; pulses not palpable in lower extremities, but capillary perfusion appears adequate. Musculoskeletal: mild flexion contractures in upper extremities; more resistance to flexion in lower extremities, with extensive tone about hips in particular; hamstrings tight; stance crouched, with valgus feet and hallux valgus; spine straight. Neurologic: reflexes symmetrically brisk.

Laboratory Findings: Electrolytes normal, serum albumin 4.4 g/dl, total protein 7.3 g/dl. Chest x-rays, EKG, echocardiogram, and abdominal ultrasound: normal. Urinalysis and CBC: normal. Liver function and renal function tests: normal; euthyroid. Rheumatoid factor and ANA: negative. Karyotype: normal, 46 XX. Radionuclide lymphangiogram (see figure): marked delay in uptake bilaterally—nearly an hour to visualize on left; never really seen on right, although tracer eventually appeared in right pelvic nodes. Extremities: serial measurements of legs diminished by 3–4 cm with sequential compression pumping; upper extremity edema attributed to dependency and better support needed in sitting and gait activities.

Question: Is this presentation consistent with typical lymphedema praecox (idiopathic lymphedema due to congenital lymphatic abnormality, first becoming evident around puberty)?

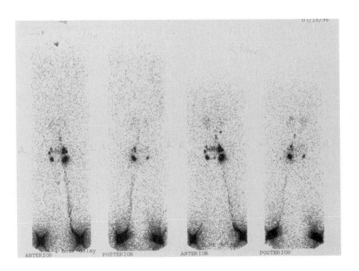

Answer: No, these symptoms represent a combination of medication-induced edema and lipedema.

Discussion: The patient's abnormal lymphangiogram demonstrated marked delay in uptake in the lymphatic channels bilaterally, more so on the right than the left. Her baclofen was increased to 10 mg TID to try to reduce spasticity, but on follow-up, she also had facial edema and an additional 5-kg weight gain. Lower extremities had not improved further despite adherence to the treatment protocol. Other explanations for her difficulties were sought.

In idiopathic lymphedema, the lymphatic structures are actually congenitally absent, and usually only the lower extremities are involved. Weaning baclofen provided quick resolution of the facial and upper extremity edema over the next few weeks, but significant lower extremity edema persisted. An MRI scan of the affected extremity can differentiate between lymphedema and a related condition called lipedema, which is basically a functional obstruction to lymphatic drainage, occurring in obese individuals. It relatively spares feet and ankles, in this case not as obviously probably due to the component of medication-related edema.

In the present patient, an MRI scan (see figure below) showed marked atrophy of lower extremity musculature, with prominence of superficial and deep fatty tissues, but no "honeycomb" pattern and no edema in the muscular tissues as would be expected in lymphedema. She has since stabilized her weight at 80–85 kg. Ground-reaction ankle-foot orthoses are again usable despite some swelling and hamstring tightness, and she again walks short distances with her walker. The patient also uses a power wheelchair, as she has gone on to college and is academically doing very well. This combination of related factors producing edema—medication side effect, decreased ambulation, and marked weight gain associated with lipedema—required careful consideration of possible rare medication side effects and an amended diagnosis to stop its progression.

Daily sequential compression pumping is a time-consuming procedure. It was only partially effective for this condition, though very effective and appropriate for true lymphedema of the upper and lower extremities. The frequency of pumping was gradually reduced, and is now used on an as-needed basis.

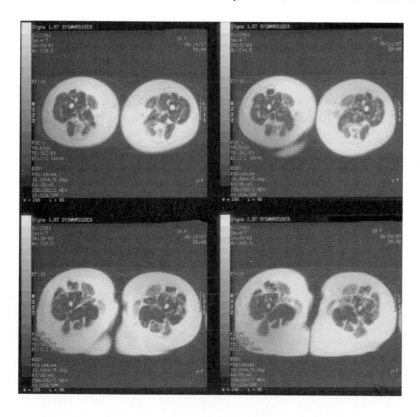

Clinical Pearls

1. Always consider medication side effects, especially if increasing the dosage makes symptoms worse.

2. Be diligent with your diagnostic evaluations. If the working diagnosis doesn't quite fit, look for others—especially when treatment fails.

3. When traditional diagnostic studies are non-diagnostic, consider others. MRI and CT are valuable in unusual circumstances.

REFERENCES

1. Beninson J, Edelglass JW: Lipedema—the non-lymphatic masquerader. Angiology 35(8):506–510, 1984.
2. Duewell S, Hagspiel KD, Zuber J, et al: Swollen lower extremity: Role of MR imaging. Radiology 184(1):227–231, 1992.
3. Hadjis NS, Carr DH, Banks L, Pflug JJ: The role of CT in the diagnosis of primary lymphedema of the lower limb. Am J Roentgenol 144(2): 361–364, 1985.
4. Schmitz R: Lipedema from the differential diagnostic and therapeutic viewpoint. [translated from German] Z Hautkr 62(2):146–157, 1987.
5. Weissleder H, Brauer JW, Schuchhardt C, Herpertz U: Value of functional lymphoscintigraphy and indirect lymphangiography in lipedema syndrome. [translated from German] Z Lymphol 19(2):38–41, 1995.
6. Young JR: The swollen leg. Am Fam Physician 15(1):163–173, 1977.

PATIENT 51

A 36-year-old man with a spinal cord injury and abnormal urodynamics

A 36-year-old man with a history of a C6 complete spinal cord injury 1 year ago reports no problems with bladder management. His wife performs clean intermittent catheterization every 6 hours at home. He reports the volumes of the in/out catheterization are about 200–300 cc. He has had one urinary tract infection in the last year. He noticed the urine smelled foul, but denied any symptoms of fever, incontinence, or chills. The infection cleared after treatment with oral antibiotics. He returns to your clinic for routine follow-up. You arrange for routine urodynamics with the urologist. The patient's medications are: baclofen 20 mg po QID; Axid 150 mg po BID; diazepam 5 mg po TID; Colace 100 mg BID; Allegra 60 mg po BID.

Physical Examination: Temperature 98.2°; pulse 62; respiration 16; blood pressure 102/72. HEENT: normal. Chest: clear. Cardiac: normal. Abdomen: soft, with normal active bowel sound. Musculoskeletal: normal range of motion in upper and lower extremities, except contractures developing in proximal and distal interphalangeal joints of both hands. Neurologic: cranial nerves II–XII intact; 3+ knee jerks bilaterally; sustained clonus in both ankle; positive Hoffmann sign bilaterally; positive Babinski sign bilaterally; absent light touch and pinprick sensation below C6 dermatome, bilaterally; absence of proprioception in both lower extremities; normal strength in upper extremities with shoulder abduction and elbow flexion; 4+/5 strength with right wrist extension and 4/5 strength with left wrist extension; 0/5 strength with elbow extension, finger flexion, and abduction of the little finger, bilaterally; 0/5 strength in lower extremities, bilaterally. Rectal: no sensation to light touch, pinprick, and pressure sensation; no voluntary anal contraction; positive bulbocavernous reflex. Skin: normal.

Laboratory Findings: WBC 6400/μl; hct 39%; platelets 203,000/μl. aspartate aminotransferase 14 U/L; alanine aminotransferase 12 U/L; albumin 3.2 g/dl; BUN 20 mg/dl; creatinine 0.7 mg/dl. Urinalysis: yellow and slightly cloudy; pH 6.5; specific gravity 1.025; protein, blood, nitrate, leukocyte esterase negative; trace bacteria; occasional WBC/hpf. Renal ultrasound: normal kidney size, no evidence of hydronephrosis, normal renal cortex. Spinal MRI: good anterior fixation and spinal alignment; no evidence of syringomyelia. Urodynamics: bladder pressures 25–45 cm of water (see figure).

Question: What does the cystogram below show? What is your diagnosis?

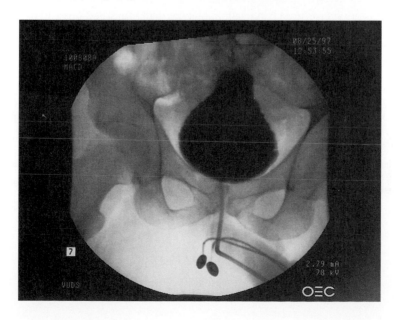

Answer: Bladder wall trabeculation with "Christmas tree effect," consistent with detrusor hyperreflexia.

Discussion: This patient was performing clean intermittent catheterizations four times a day with low bladder volumes. He was quite content with his bladder management and had no complaints. However, on routine urodynamics significant bladder wall hypertrophy and trabeculations were noted despite bladder pressures that were not that high. This suggests persistent elevated bladder pressures and loss of bladder compliance that is asymptomatic. The urodynamic study was the only way to find out early on that he was having trouble and intervene to prevent later complications.

Mortality from renal failure has decreased markedly in the last decades. This is probably due to many factors, including improved materials in appliances and indwelling catheters, other methods for management of bladder drainage, greater attention and monitoring of bladder management, and improved antibiotics. In this patient the high-pressure bladder system must be controlled or the urinary deterioration will eventually lead to renal deterioration. Oral antimuscarinic agents, such as oxybutynin or the newer tolterodine, can be used; however, they can cause the intolerable side effects of dry mouth and constipation. Intravesical instillation of oxybutynin can be done after each catheterization. Capsaicin can be infused into the bladder by the urologist for refractory detrusor hyperreflexia.

Other methods of bladder management to prevent chronic bladder pressure elevation should also be discussed with the patient. Since he is having good success and is happy with intermittent catheterization, antimuscarinic medication should be tried first. If it is unsuccessful, an indwelling Foley catheter could be tried, but the risk of bladder bacterial colonization is virtually 100%. Surgical options consist of the following:

1. External sphincterotomy and use of a condom catheter with a leg bag

2. Suprapubic catheter with a leg bag

3. Augmentation cystoplasty, with a continent stoma, with continued intermittent catheterizations

4. Augmentation cystoplasty with an appendicovesicostomy. The appendix is brought to the umbilicus to create a tube to catheterize the bladder via the umbilicus.

5. Sacral root dorsal rhizotomy to allow the bladder to expand, along with a sacral root electrical stimulator to empty the bladder.

6. Ileovesicostomy, in which the ileum is attached to the top of the bladder, like a chimney, and is connected to the skin. This allows urine to drain from the bladder, promoting low bladder pressures.

Since the present patient was having no problems with in/out catheterization, he was started on high-dose oxybutynin. His bladder compliance and pressures improved. However, the patient desired to return to school and did not want to have to have someone catheterize him every 6 hours, so he elected to have a suprapubic catheter. He is doing well with the suprapubic catheter and is now attending classes successfully with increased independence.

Clinical Pearls

1. Detrusor hyperreflexia can result in bladder wall trabeculations and hypertrophy.
2. A high-pressure bladder system can cause reflux and renal deterioration.
3. There are many ways to manage detrusor hyperreflexia, and the patient and physician should decide together which option is best.

REFERENCES

1. Brendler C, Radebaugh B, Lisa C, Mohler J: Topical oxybutynin chloride for relaxation of dysfunctional bladder. J Urol 144:270–273, 1990.
2. Brindley GS: The first 500 patients with sacral anterior root stimulator implants: general description. Paraplegia 32: 795–805, 1994.
3. Lazzeri M, Spinelli M, Beneforti P, et al: Urodynamic assessment during intravesical infusion of capsaicin for the treatment of refractory detrusor hyperreflexia. Spinal Cord 37: 440–443, 1999.
4. Stover SL, Lloyd KL, Waites KB, Jackson AB: Urinary tract infection in spinal cord injury. Arch Phys Med Rehabil 70:47–54, 1989.

PATIENT 52

A 69-year-old woman with low back and leg pain
after pruning a fruit tree

A 69-year-old woman presents for evaluation of low back and leg pain of 4-month duration. Three days prior to the onset of her symptoms she had spent 2 hours working in her yard pruning a fruit tree. She initially developed only lower back pain, but by the second day, the pain began to radiate down into the right thigh and leg. Currently, sitting and bending relieve the pain. When shopping, she gets relief by resting forward on the shopping cart. Standing longer than 2 minutes and walking longer than 5 minutes brings on her pain. She has a prior history of osteoporosis with a remote T8 compression fracture. Her current medications include ibuprofen, nasal calcitonin, estrogen supplementation, and multivitamins.

Physical Examination: General: in moderate distress; ambulating in a forward flexed posture without evidence of antalgia or other gait disturbance. Spine: no evidence of postural or scoliotic deformity. Musculoskeletal: tenderness in ower right lumbar paraspinal segments and right sciatic notch region; limited lumbar extension reproduces back and leg symptoms. Neurologic: reflexes symmetric and sensation intact throughout; 4/5- dorsiflexor weakness in right foot; no evidence of atrophy or fasciculation; Trendelenberg and SLR tests negative bilaterally; peripheral pulses intact 1+ bilaterally at popliteal and posterior tibial sites.

Laboratory Findings: Plain films of pelvis: normal. Plain films of lumbar spine: localized degenerative disc disease at L4/5, 10% anterior wedging deformity of L1, and diffuse demineralization.

Question: What is causing this patient's back and leg pain?

Diagnosis: Degenerative lumbar spinal stenosis with acute neurogenic claudication

Discussion: Degenerative lumbar spinal stenosis (LSS) as a clinical entity can be described as any narrowing of the lumbar spinal canal with resultant signs and symptoms due to secondary compression of vascular and neural tissues. The term implies that the spinal canal narrowing is not primarily discogenic in nature (i.e., not caused by disc herniation).

The most common factor in the development of LSS is **disc degeneration** and the **hypertrophic changes** that accompany it. Gross features of the stenotic spine include a thickened lamina, hypertrophic facet joints, thickened ligamentum flavum, narrowed lateral recesses, and neural foramen. Other contributing factors include disc herniation, spondylolisthesis, congenital spinal narrowing, Paget's disease, synovial cysts, scoliosis, and achondroplasia.

The cardinal symptom complex in the LSS patient is **neurogenic claudication**. This describes the pattern of pain and/or paresthesias in the back and legs, which is brought on by standing and walking and relieved by sitting or flexing the lumbar spine. In contrast to vascular claudication, the stenosis patient may be symptomatic with simple standing and may not have leg symptoms when riding a bicycle. Dynamic reduction in the cross-sectional area for the dura occurs as the lumbar spine moves from flexion to extension, therein providing a biomechanical explanation for the symptom complex.

The clinical course of LSS is one of chronic symptoms of back and radicular pain: 70% of untreated patients have no change in symptoms, 15% improve, and 15% worsen over time. In patients treated conservatively, fair to excellent results have been reported in 50% followed over 10 years. Long-term nonsurgical treatment did not result in clinically significant deterioration in symptoms. Surgical outcomes were similar for those patients electing initially to pursue conservative care. Surgical results have been described as favorable in most studies. Long-term follow-up in surgically treated patients has clearly shown favorable results in the majority of patients studied.

The diagnosis is made on clinical and radiographic bases. The majority of patients present with atypical leg pain that does not follow any particular radicular pattern. Back pain is commonly associated with the leg symptoms. Once the patient clinically fulfills the criteria for neurogenic claudication, the clinician confirms the diagnosis with radiographic studies. Currently, **MRI** is the most common diagnostic procedure used in the assessment of LSS. Due to the superior ability to visualize subtle bony hypertrophy on **CT with myelography**, it is considered the gold standard in diagnostic imaging for this condition. Physical examination is usually unremarkable. A severely symptomatic patient may present with a forward flexed posture while walking toward or standing in the exam room.

Little is published on the conservative management of this condition. The typical conservative treatment plan includes avoidance of aggravating activities; physical therapy referral to develop a comprehensive flexion-biased home exercise program; pharmacologic control of pain and inflammation; and a trial of lumbar epidural steroid injections (ESIs). Transforaminal ESIs have been shown to be clinically safe with low incidence of complications. In the more symptomatic patients, surgical decompression usually provides satisfactory results.

The present patient demonstrated acute symptoms of right L5 radiculopathy following a pattern of neurogenic claudication. Based upon the severity of her symptoms an MRI of the lumbar spine was ordered (see figure). It revealed severe localized spinal stenosis at the degenerative L4/5 level. Her pattern of right L5 radicular pain is explained by compression of the fifth lumbar nerve root in the lateral recess. Electrodiagnostic studies were not performed. She was given NSAIDs for pain control and referred to physical therapy for modalities and therapeutic exercise. Due to persistent disabling radicular pain, a transforaminal ESI at the right L5-S1 level was performed with excellent response. Upon discharge, the patient was counseled regarding avoidance of aggravating activities as well as performance of a routine home exercise program.

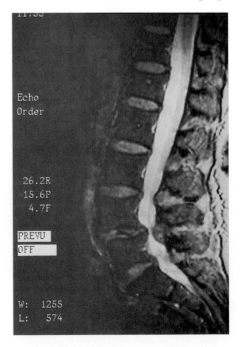

Clinical Pearls

1. Neurogenic claudication is a clinical hallmark of lumbar spinal stenosis and is characterized by reproduction of radicular pain with activities that induce lumbar lordosis, typically standing and walking. Those symptoms are usually relieved by flexion-based activities such as sitting and bending.

2. Physical examination is usually unremarkable for localizing neurologic deficit.

3. Conservative management is advisable and is unlikely to result in neurologic deterioration.

4. For patients in whom conservative treatment fails, surgical outcomes are usually favorable.

5. Despite radiographic evidence of advanced spinal stenosis, patients may remain asymptomatic for years until a biomechanical trauma or perturbation occurs.

REFERENCES

1. Amundsen T, Weber H, et al: Lumbar spinal stenosis: conservative or surgical management? A Prospective 10-year Study. Spine 25: 1424–1436, 2000.
2. Hanley EN Jr: The surgical treatment of lumbar degenerative disease. In Garfin SR, Vaccaro AR (eds): Orthopedic Knowledge Update: Spine. Rosemont, Illinois, American Academy of Orthopedic Surgeons, 1997, pp 130–133.
3. Johnsson KE, Rosen I, Uden A: The natural course of lumbar spinal stenosis. Clin Orthop 279:82–86, 1992.

PATIENT 53

A 46-year-old man with a history of right below-knee amputation

A 46-year-old man with a history of right below-knee amputation presents with dry skin and painful eruptions on the distal part of his stump. His injury was sustained in a blast injury at an oil refinery where he was a supervisor, and he has been a successful prosthetic user for the past 10 years. The patient's current symptoms developed several months ago. Treatment has consisted of topical antibiotic ointment and cortisone preparations, with little improvement. The patient also reports a 3-month history of mild edema and some redness of the distal stump. There has been no revision of his prosthetic socket in over 5 years. He currently uses a patella tendon-bearing socket with a P-lite liner, with fewer stump socks than in the past. He is an active and ambulatory—in fact, he is employed at the refinery where his initial injury occurred. The patient estimates that he walks up to three miles a day in his current job position.

The patient's past medical history is negative for heart disease and diabetes. He has mild hypertension, which is controlled with lisinopril 20 mg po q day. He does not smoke, and drinks alcohol only occasionally.

Physical Examination: General: well developed, non-obese, no acute distress. Cardiac: regular rate and rhythm, without murmur. Chest: clear to auscultation. Musculoskeletal: stump length 22 cm; mild bulbous deformity with nonpitting edema over anterior tibial surface. Skin: scaling; two separate 1 cm x 1 cm ulcerations, healing well; slightly dry, with leathery texture. Quadriceps muscle strength is 5/5. No flexion contracture noted in the knee. Gait: normal alignment of prosthesis in residual limb; reciprocal with equal stride lengths; no excessive hip circumduction or hip-hike.

Laboratory Findings: CBC normal, WBC 7000/μl, electrolytes and ESR normal.

Questions: What is the patient's skin condition? What is the likely cause?

Answer: Verrucous hyperplasia due to inadequate total contact of the prosthetic socket.

Discussion: The consideration of socket design in a patient with transtibial amputation is very important and should be tailored to the specific patient. Complications can arise due to inadequate contact with the intact stump, leading to malformation, especially early in the post-amputation phase. During this phase, significant changes occur in the residual stump, and care should be taken to avoid bulbous end deformities. These are often due to a choking phenomenon, in which the proximal portion of the socket is tight, and distal contact is poor. As the stump matures, however, volume changes are less dramatic. This discussion centers on the most common types of socket design in the transtibial amputee.

The socket portion of the prosthesis in a patient with transtibial amputation is the interface by which body weight is transmitted through the residual limb during ambulation as well as stance. Proper fit is of paramount importance to decrease shear and offer maximal biomechanical advantage. Certain anatomic areas of the residual limb have been described as more pressure tolerant than others. More pressure-tolerant areas include the medial tibial flair, lateral tibial flair, anterior compartment muscle, and patella tendon. Relatively intolerant areas include the distal tibia, fibular head, and tibial tubercle. Historically, socket design has been directed at maximizing the use of pressure-tolerant areas.

The **patella tendon-bearing socket**, introduced in the late 1950s, is the most commonly used design. It incorporates the total contact theory for weight bearing, in which specific weight-tolerant and intolerant areas of the residual limb are identified, and the biomechanics are defined for each phase of gait. This theory includes the application of some contact to the distal end of the residual stump, which had previously been thought to need significant relief. Anterior and posterior shifting is reduced through counter pressure from the posterior wall of the socket by the gastrocnemius, while rotational control is added by the anterior compartment musculature. Weight bearing over the fibular shaft functions as a counter force to the anterior lateral force directed against the medial tibial flair, resulting in lateral stabilization. Weight-intolerant areas are usually avoided by relief grooves of the sockets.

Two modifications have been developed to increase medial lateral stability of the patella tendon-bearing socket: the supracondylar design and the supracondylar-suprapatellar design. These designs do offer some biomechanical advantage; however, they are often found cosmetically unacceptable as they extend above the surface of the knee in flexion.

Another type of component, the **total surface-bearing socket**, is based on the theory that the pressure should be distributed more equally across the entire surface of the residual limb. Areas that were previously felt to be intolerant to weight are incorporated into weight bearing. The interface material used in the liner of the socket is critical in this mechanism. Popular liner materials incorporate urethane, mineral oil gel, or silicone. Their main advantage is the ability to deal with multidirectional shear forces, thus increasing total surface contact and reducing skin compromise. Total surface-bearing sockets are especially good for patients who have had skin grafting or have excessive scar tissue. The liners also tend to have shock-absorbing properties and can be beneficial in patients who have a short residual or a conical-shaped limb.

A third socket design is referred to as a **hydrostatic socket**. It incorporates Pascal's principle of fluid dynamics. The principle is that pressure on any surface exerts a force perpendicular to that surface. Thus, in this mechanism no certain portion of the residual limb is identified as needing more or less weight bearing; pressure is equally transmitted to the overall limb soft tissue. This type of socket requires careful application of a pressure casting system by a prosthetist to obtain an accurate plaster mold. One drawback to this design is that it does not account for the different biomechanical weight-bearing changes that occur during the gait cycle. The hydrostatic socket is to be used in combination with a silicone suspension system and liner.

In writing prescriptions for the transtibial amputee, consider the patient's overall medical condition, the condition of the limb, and the anticipated level of activity. Optimal function is achieved through proper socket design, suspension, and alignment with the proper prosthetic foot.

Clinical Pearls

1. The socket design used most frequently by the below-knee amputee is the patella tendon-bearing socket.

2. Total surface-bearing theories have led to the development of new socket liners that reduce shear and friction on the skin of the residual limb.

3. Hydrostatic socket design depends on pressure and fluid dynamics distributed in a uniform manner. Pressure casting is necessary to mold the residual limb uniformly.

REFERENCES

1. Ferguson J, Smith DG: Socket considerations for the patient with a transtibial amputation. Clin Orthopaed Rel Res 361:76–84, 1999.
2. Shurr DG, Cook TM: Prosthetics and Orthotics. Stamford, CT, Appleton and Lange, 1990.

PATIENT 54

A 65-year-old woman with muscle aches and stiffness

A 65-year-old woman presents with a 6-month history of generalized muscle aches and stiffness. It has become increasingly difficult for her to find the energy to maintain her daily home and outside chores. Several days ago, she started to have difficulty with balance while walking, and actually fell on two occasions; fortunately she suffered only minor abrasions. Her sister, with whom she shares a home, has noticed that she "seems depressed." The patient has a history of mild hypertension, non-insulin-dependent diabetes mellitus, and hypothyroidism (stable). She is on medications for all three conditions.

Physical Examination: Vital signs: stable. General: alert, but with flat affect. Neurologic: oriented to person, place, and situation; immediate recall of three objects normal, but 3-minute recall abnormal (only one object remembered); cranial nerves 2–12 grossly intact, including visual fields; sensory and motor normal; 1+ reflexes in all extremities. Musculoskeletal: mild rigidity in all extremities; gait has narrow base of support, with short stride lengths. Cardiac, chest, and abdomen: normal.

Question: How would you explain this patient's flat affect?

Answer: Masked facial expression associated with Parkinson's disease

Discussion: Parkinson's disease (PD) is a movement disorder entailing degeneration of nuclei in the basal ganglia, especially the substantia nigra. Normally, neurons based in the substantia nigra facilitate movement by releasing dopamine into the striatum, but in PD dopamine production and release is reduced. The etiology is not certain, but some theoretical causes are environmental toxins, accelerated aging, genetic predisposition, and oxidative stress.

The signs and symptoms of PD include rigidity, resting or postural tremor, bradykinesia, and postural instability. Masked facies and bradykinesia lead to the most common misdiagnosis of depression. Cognitive deficits and dementia are often present. Those with rigidity as the major early sign tend to develop disability earlier than people with tremor as the presenting feature. As the disease advances, autonomic instability occurs.

The gold-standard treatment for PD is **oral dopaminergic medications** such as carbidopa-levodopa, bromocriptine, and selegiline. These medications help to restore function, but they do have side effects, including insomnia, hallucinations, lack of appetite, and dystonia.

Until recently, most studies revealed few lasting benefits of rehabilitation for people with PD. Most of the emphasis has been on maintaining function and compensatory-energy conservation strategies. Recent studies show that **external sensory cues** result in significant improvement in motor function and ability to resume activities of daily living (ADLs) in moderate PD. Moreover, auditory cues have been shown to improve execution of motor sequences. Music therapy has produced improved movement patterns, emotional stability, ADL capacity, and quality of life. The theory behind the benefits of auditory cues and music therapy is that external cues help to replace defective internally generated discharges of the basal ganglia.

The present patient took part in a 4-week comprehensive rehabilitation program incorporating physical and occupational therapies, speech therapy, and psychological treatment. Physical therapy focused on her posture, balance, proper weight shifting, fall prevention, and gait training using auditory and visual cues. Occupational therapy worked on ADLs and energy conservation, and a home evaluation was performed for environmental safety and adaptive equipment. Speech therapy worked on variation of speech quality and volume as well as facial expressions. Her medical management was orchestrated by her physiatrist and neurologist. She was able to adhere to her home exercises by joining a PD group for both exercise and socialization.

Clinical Pearls

1. The most common misdiagnosis in Parkinson's disease (PD) is depression, which is based on the PD symptoms of masked facies and bradykinesia.

2. Those with rigidity as the presenting feature tend to develop disability earlier than those with tremor as the initial feature.

3. Traditionally, full-team rehabilitation has not resulted in lasting improvements in the function of PD patients; however, recent studies suggest that external cues in the form of auditory, visual, and sensory stimuli can have long-term benefits for function in PD.

4. PD patients who have made functional gains in rehabilitation tend to decline back to baseline if they do not adhere to the exercises and strategies that were taught in the rehabilitation program.

5. While dopaminergic agents are the gold-standard treatment for PD, a number of side effects directly result from the boost in this neurotransmitter.

REFERENCES

1. Comella CL, Stebbins GT, Brown-Tom SN, Goetz CG: Physical therapy and Parkinson's disease: A controlled clinical trial. Neurology 44(1):376–378, 1994.
2. Kritikos A, Leahy C, Bradshaw JL, Iansek R, et al: Contingent and non-contingent auditory cueing in PD. Neuropsychologia 33(10): 1193–1203, 1995.
3. Dombovy ML: Rehabilitation concerns in degenerative movement disorders of the central nervous system. In Braddom RL (ed): Physical Medicine and Rehabilitation. Philadelphia, WB Saunders Co, 1996, pp 1088–1112.
4. Pacchetti C, Mancini F, Aglieri R, Fundaro C, et al: Active music therapy in PD: An integrative method for motor and emotional rehabilitation. Psychosom Med 62(3): 386–393, 2000.
5. Marchese R, Diverio M, Zucchi F, Lentino C, et al: The role of sensory cues in the rehabilitation of parkinsonian patients: A comparison of two physical therapy protocols. Movement Disorder 15(5): 879–883, 2000.

PATIENT 55

A 36-year-old man with traumatic brain injury and the acute onset of emotional distress

A 36-year-old man presents following a severe traumatic brain injury as the result of a motor vehicle accident. Associated injuries included a right brachial plexopathy documented by EMG and nerve conduction studies. He successfully completed an inpatient rehabilitation program and was discharged to independent living. Approximately 3 months after his initial injury, he enrolled in an outpatient neurorehabilitation program under the supervision of a neuropsychologist. When he complained of continued burning pain in a distribution consistent with his neuropathy despite acetaminophen, ibuprofen, and use of transcutaneous electrical nerve stimulation (TENS), he was started on gabapentin, 300 mg PO three times daily, for treatment of neuropathic pain. In addition, ibuprofen, acetaminophen, and codeine were given at increasingly higher doses to address the patient's pain complaints. Within 1 week, the patient reported acute emotional distress, consisting of heightened anxiety and psychomotor restlessness.

The patient's past medical history is noncontributory. There is a family history of bipolar disorder in his mother.

Physical Examination: Mental status: alert, oriented, and aware of reason for admission; able to perform "serial sevens," name three objects after 5 minutes, and recall the past three U.S. presidents. Motor exam: visible repetitive movements during the exam—toe-tapping, fidgeting, and difficulty remaining seated. Sensory exam: increased sensitivity to light touch; intolerance to pin-prick testing in distribution of right median nerve.

Question: What is the cause of the patient's acute emotional distress?

Answer: Gabapentin

Discussion: This case illustrates psychomotor symptoms related to ingestion of gabapentin. While other agents used to treat the patient's pain complaints might also be suspected of adverse effects, the patient's emotional distress and restlessness dramatically improved within 48 hours of discontinuation of gabapentin.

In long-term studies in both animal and humans, gabapentin had a favorable toxicity profile, no known anti-epileptic drug interactions, no active metabolites, and a 5- to 7-hour elimination half-life. In clinical studies, most adverse effects are dose dependent and generally resolve following discontinuation of the drug. Approximately 7% of 2074 individuals given gabapentin in premarketing trials discontinued treatment because of an adverse event. The most common events were somnolence, dizziness, ataxia, and fatigue. Nervousness was reported as an adverse event only slightly more frequently (2.4%) than placebo (1.9%).

In the present patient, nervousness was equated to findings of heightened anxiety and psychomotor restlessness.

Clinical Pearls

1. Physicians treating brain-injured patients and prescribing gabapentin for neuropathic pain should closely monitor patients for signs of restlessness or anxiety.

2. In any patient with a history of brain trauma or psychiatric problems, proceed with caution when initiating agents that have a potential to alter mood or state of mind. No brain injury is alike, and responses may vary widely among individuals.

REFERENCES
1. Berker E: Diagnosis, physiology, pathology and rehabilitation of traumatic brain injuries. Int J Neurosci 85:195–220, 1996.
2. Beydoun A, Uthman BM, Sackellares JC: Gabapentin: Pharmacokinetics, efficacy, and safety. Clin Neuropharmacol 18:469–481, 1995.
3. Childers MK, Holland D: Psychomotor agitation following gabapentin use in brain injury. Brain Injury 11:537–540, 1997.
4. Kelly KM: Gabapentin. Antiepileptic mechanism of action. Neuropsychobiology 38:139–144, 1998.

PATIENT 56

A 72-year old-woman with aching muscles and difficulty rising

A 72-year old-woman complains of difficulty rising from a chair and vague aching in her muscles beginning 4 months prior to the evaluation. You observe that she uses her hands to rise from a chair and pulls herself to standing from a squat by using her hands on the examining table.

Physical Examination: Extremities: mild proximal weakness in both legs (5-/5 in bilateral hip flexors); normal strength in arms. Gait: unremarkable, with no evidence of abnormality such as "waddling." Neurologic: deep tendon reflexes and sensory exam normal.

Laboratory Findings: Serum CPK: increased four-fold. See results of nerve conduction and EMG studies below.

Question: What is the cause of this woman's difficulties?

Nerve Conduction Study

Nerve	Site	Latency	NCV	Amplitude	F wave
R median (m)	Wrist-APB	3.8 ms		10.50 mv	26.7 ms
	Elbow-wrist		55.7 m/s	9.90 mv	
R peroneal (m)	Ankle-EDB	4.6 ms		4.4 mv	52.0 ms
	FH-ankle		40.8 m/s	3.30 mv	
R sural (s)	Calf-lat mal	NR			
R median (s)	Dig III-wrist	2.0 ms	64.0 m/s	40.80μV	

(m) = motor, (s) = sensory, NCV = nerve conduction velocity, APB = abductor pollicis brevis, EDB = extensor digitorum brevis, FH = fibular head

EMG Study

Muscle	Fibs	PSWs	Fascic	MUAP duration	MUAP amplitude	MUAP morph.	Interfer Pattern
R deltoid	0	0	0	Nl	Nl	Nl	Full
R vastus med	1+	1+	0	Brief	Nl	Nl	Enhanced
R vastus lat	2+	2+	0	Brief	Nl	Polyphasic	Enhanced
Right tib ant	0	0	0	Nl	Nl	Nl	Full

PSW = positive sharp waves, MUAP = motor unit action potential, Nl = normal

Diagnosis: Polymyositis

Discussion: Nerve conduction studies are normal for this patient's age, since an absent sural sensory nerve action potential (SNAP) may be found in a 72-year-old patient without any associated pathology. Nerve conduction studies are typically normal in myopathies; although if the weakness is severe, motor nerve compound muscle action potential (CMAP) amplitudes may be reduced. In this case, the EMG needle examination shows evidence for a mild acute deinnervation in the vastus muscles. Motor unit action potentials (MUAP) in these muscles are brief, with some polyphasic morphology and normal amplitudes. MUAPs with this appearance are consistent with a myopathic process.

In myopathies, muscle fibers are lost or atrophic and may vary in size; all of these pathologic features of a myopathy contribute to the changes found in the MUAP. The acute denervation changes are typically seen with disorders such as polymyositis that involve muscle fiber degeneration. Other myopathies in which both MUAP changes and fibrillation potentials can be found are **inclusion body myositis**, **dermatomyositis**, and **muscular dystrophy**.

Following treatment and/or clinical remission, the fibrillation potentials in polymyositis are typically lost, although the MUAP changes can persist. The enhanced interference pattern seen in this patient is related to the central nervous system recognizing that the force generated in the muscle is insufficient for the number of motor units firing. The central nervous system compensates by increasing the number of motor units that are firing, as well as increasing their firing rate.

In polymyositis, the abnormal findings on EMG are frequently patchy, so some muscles may be normal while others are abnormal. Proximal muscles of the extremities and the paraspinal muscles are particularly likely to be abnormal in polymyositis. Selection of muscles on which to perform the EMG needle exam is prudently based on discovering the weakest ones on clinical exam. If the EMG changes are predominantly found in the distal musculature, the diagnosis of inclusion body myositis should be entertained. Clinically, a patient with inclusion body myositis has a more chronic course, only mildly elevated CPK, and weakness typically in the wrist and finger flexors, quadriceps, and foot dorsiflexors.

Clinical Pearls

1. Short-duration MUAPs are the most sensitive indicator of a myopathy. While reduced amplitude of the MUAPs can also be found, it reflects only the few muscles fibers that are in close proximity to the electrode and is, therefore, less sensitive.

2. The degree of fibrillation present tends to correlate with disease activity in polymyositis.

3. Although brief, small-amplitude, polyphasic MUAPs are typical for a myopathy, they can also be found in other disorders including Guillain Barré syndrome (because of conduction block) and Lambert Eaton myasthenic syndrome (because of neuromuscular transmission block).

4. In end-stage muscle disease, recruitment of motor units is often reduced because muscle has been replaced with fatty and connective tissue. This replacement of active muscle tissue produces a firing pattern that appears neurogenic.

REFERENCES
1. Bromberg MD, Albers JW: Electromyography in idiopathic myositis. Mt Sinai J Med 55(6):459-464, 1988.
2. Mechler F: Changing electromyographic findings during the chronic course of polymyositis. J Neurol Sci 23:237-242, 1974.
3. Robinson LR: AAEM Case report #22: Polymyositis. Muscle and Nerve 14:310-315, 1991.
4. Wilburn AJ: The electrodiagnostic examination with myopathies. J Clin Neurophysiol 10:132-148, 1993.

PATIENT 57

A 19-year-old man with traumatic brain injury and quadriplegia

A 19-year-old man has a traumatic brain injury from an accident in which he was hit by a car while walking across the street. He was initially comatose. No spinal cord injury was found. After his stay in an acute care hospital, he is transferred to a transitional care facility. He is observed to have sleep-wake cycles and frequent periods of alertness. He has a gastrostomy tube, but no tracheostomy.

Physical Examination: Blood pressure 125/70, pulse 99, respiration 20, temperature 98°. General: awake and alert; thin; no distress or agitation; visual tracking noted. Neurologic: patient was able to follow commands using eye and head movements, but was completely aphonic; sensory testing difficult because of aphonia, but generalized withdrawal responses exhibited to strong tactile and painful stimuli. Musculoskeletal: 0/5 muscle strength in upper and lower extremities; spasticity in all limbs, rated 2 on modified Ashworth scale.

Question: What syndrome does this patient have?

Diagnosis: Locked-in syndrome

Discussion: Locked-in syndrome is defined by the American Congress of Rehabilitation Medicine as "a specific neurobehavioral diagnosis that refers to patients who are alert, cognitively aware of their environment, and capable of communication, but cannot move or speak." The following are the neurobehavioral criteria for the syndrome:

• Well-sustained eye opening (bilateral ptosis needs to be ruled out if a patient cannot open his/her eyes, but demonstrates eye movement when the eyelids are opened manually)
• Basic cognitive abilities
• Clinical evidence of severe hypophonia or aphonia
• Clinical evidence of quadriparesis or quadriplegia
• Primary mode of communication is vertical or lateral eye movements or blinking.

Lesions in bilateral ventral pontine areas cause this syndrome, most commonly from infarction. The lesions interrupt the pathways found in bilateral corticospinal and corticobulbar tracts.

Once diagnosed, strategies for effective communication with a patient who has locked-in syndrome vary from simple mouthpieces to computer programs using laser pointers. Doble et al. studied the quality of life of 29 such patients. At the end of 11 years, 14 patients were still alive, and only one expressed a wish to die. Most of the rest of the survivors participated in family life, and continued to enjoy some quality of life.

Clinical Pearls

1. The triad of preserved consciousness, quadriplegia/quadriparesis, and hypophonia/aphonia characterizes locked-in syndrome.
2. Lesions in bilateral pons, usually from infarcts, are responsible for the syndrome.
3. In patients with bilateral ptosis, manual lifting of both eyelids is necessary to determine the presence or absence of volitional eye movements.

REFERENCES

1. American Congress of Rehabilitation Medicine: Recommendations for use of uniform nomenclature pertinent to patients with severe alterations in consciousness. Position paper. Arch Phys Med Rehabil 76:205–209, 1995.
2. Doble JE, Anderson C, Haig AJ, Katz RT: Functional and quality of life issues of 29 locked-in syndrome patients followed for 11 years. Arch Phys Med Rehabil 78:1022, 1997.
3. Roth EJ: Stroke. In O'Young B, Young MA, Stiens SA (eds): PM&R Secrets. Philadelphia, Hanley & Belfus, 1997, pp 253–261.

PATIENT 58

A 14-year-old girl with severe juvenile rheumatoid arthritis and multiple rehabilitation problems

A 14-year-old girl was diagnosed with polyarticular juvenile rheumatoid arthritis (JRA) at the age of 2. Until age 12, she walked and attended regular school, keeping up straight A's despite fairly frequent absences. Family compliance with medications has been variable. Recently, the patient suffered two fractures: a pathological metatarsal fracture of the left foot, followed several months later by a left femur fracture sustained in a 15–20 mph frontal motor vehicle crash in which her mother injured her shoulder. She was treated with hip spica casting instead of surgical fixation because of severe osteopenia documented by densitometry measurements. Now, she is referred for inpatient rehabilitation because she did not regain any walking ability after the fractures healed.

Current medications are Miacalcin 1 puff alternating nostrils daily, sulfasalazine 250 mg BID, and Naprosyn 150 mg BID. Her medical history includes a period of prolonged oral steroid use. Her diet is poor in calcium, but she complains of heartburn with calcium supplements, so few of these have been given. During a Make-A-Wish trip to Disney World, which occurred between the two fracture events, she mainly used her wheelchair. The patient has experienced several episodes of tea-colored urine.

Stated goals of rehabilitation are to achieve weight-bearing transfers, as her mother cannot lift her, and her inaccessible home is unsuitable for a Hoyer lift, and to begin some ambulation. Expected length of stay is 2 weeks.

The patient is transported from home via ambulance and carried into the rehabilitation unit on the mattress from her bed, since she has not tolerated being transferred out of bed since her cast was removed 3 weeks prior to this admission. The family relates that the trip home after the cast removal was terrible, and she has not left her bed since she arrived home. They also reveal that she is taking a variety of narcotic pain medications.

Physical Examination: General: obvious pain; simply bumping mattress or brushing bedclothes that cover left knee causes screams. Weight: 30.1 kg. Chest: clear. Respirations: normal. Abdomen: benign, no organomegaly. Extremities: pain localized to left knee and hip; left knee effusion warm and tender; range of motion impossible both actively and passively; hips propped on pillows at 30–40° of flexion; both wrists and ankles demonstrate palpable synovial thickening and swelling. Neurologic: speech normal when pain less; cognition intact.

Laboratory Findings: Bone densitometry (performed between the two fracture events): –2.5 standard deviations total body and 0.461 g/cm² spine. Baseline (7 months prior): –1.6 and .389. After hospital stay and 6 months of Miacalcin: –1.66 and 0.430 (note that scoliosis and plate for femoral fracture made validity of these figures uncertain). Body fat: 28.4%—low lean body mass. Urinalysis: large blood and 40–45 RBC; 6–8 WBC. Culture and sensitivity: negative. ESR: 47 mm/hr (since 1994, never lower than 35, and usually in high 40s; highest recording 55). X-rays (see figures): extreme osteoporosis. Renal and liver function tests: unremarkable. Renal ultrasound: large, left, nonobstructing renal pelvic stone. Urine studies: elevation only of calcium excretion and calcium-creatinine ratio (0.55.) CBC: mild anemia; elevated platelet count. Albumin and prealbumin: low to normal.

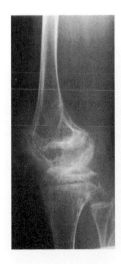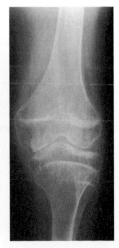

Questions: Generate a problem list and approaches to management that need to be coordinated. Are the stated rehabilitation goals of the rheumatologist and family attainable in the expected time frame?

Answer: See table for problems and approaches. The stated rehabilitation goals are *not* attainable in 2 weeks.

Discussion: The rehabilitation goals for this patient were immediately revised to pain control and portability to allow long-term outpatient therapy. Initially it was not even clear that wheelchair sitting could be attained. Nutritional rehabilitation was also undertaken, and a calcium supplement that the patient was willing to take, Viactiv, was provided, as well as preferred foods and supplements. The rehab pain team recommended regular doses of Percocet. The Percocet caused constipation, so when the patient stated that her pain was better, dosage was changed to PRN. However, this regimen kept her out of pain only as long as she did not move, which evidently had been her primary coping strategy at home. The dosage was cut in half, but administered on a regular basis, and Neurontin was added (increasing from 200 to 300 mg, then 400 mg TID), plus low-dose Ativan to address anticipatory pain reactions which gradually became apparent. A bone scan would not have been informative in regards to this therapeutic decision.

The patient received daily hydrotherapy, premedicated at first; during the first week she screamed every time her bed or stretcher was moved over a bump, but then was able to tolerate this well. She progressed to active pool therapy by discharge, but remained non-weight-bearing on land. Only active range of motion was performed, and bony fragility precautions were observed for strengthening and strength testing activities. She developed "poor plus" quadriceps strength and "fair plus" distal lower extremity strength. She maintained her antigravity to good upper extremity strength and, surprisingly, had full shoulder range of motion.

The family had been told that the patient could not do any strengthening exercises; therefore, they were educated about isometric exercise, low-resistance Theraband, and 1-pound or less weights with adapted grips that she could safely use without joint stress or injury. When expectations and prognosis were addressed, the family's and patient's sense of futility and lack of goals beyond immediate comfort if walking could not be achieved were uncovered. A psychology consultation was provided.

The head of the patient's bed was gradually raised as tolerated, and pillows were removed until she could lie flat in bed, turn herself partially, and tolerate transfers (still passive) to a reclining wheelchair. Renal workup was unrevealing except for a high urinary calcium to creatinine ratio, and diuretic therapy was begun. Azathioprine, which had been recommended and prescribed but never obtained, was added to her regimen. The family also was persuaded to try Enbrel (etanrecept) for control of her inflammation while she was still an inpatient. Her total stay was 6.5 weeks. ESR was down to 18 mm/hr at discharge.

Between discharge and follow-up, an irregular heart rate developed, and her mother admitted she was not giving her the potassium supplement with her diuretic because she complained of the taste and sometimes gagged on the one her local pharmacy

Problem List and Approaches to Management

Active JRA	Rheumatology consult, medications
Poor diet and nutrition	Nutritionist for assessment of preferences and provision of supplements, education, and encouragement
Extreme osteoporosis	Medical and nutritional treatment, since weight-bearing very limited; therapy with precautions as for osteogenesis imperfecta (active range of motion only, weight-bear in pool only, proximal hand placement and 2–3 person lifts with careful support)
Severe pain	Regular medication, both direct analgesic and for neuropathic component, sufficient to allow mobilization
Prolonged disuse and immobility	Isometric and gentle active concentric strength exercise with modified grips and interfaces
Hematuria	Work-up and treatment of hypercalcuria, per nephrology consult
Family noncompliance	Education, encouragement, psychological and peer support, and planned and serendipitous "reality therapy." (She *does* improve on consistent medication. She *could* die of hypokalemia, whether she likes her supplement or not.)
Home inaccessible	Family given information and suggestions; achieved assisted transfer without equipment

was able to supply. Hypokalemia was diagnosed, and her mother looked up the cardiac effects of hypokalemia on the Internet; after an emergency room visit and treatment for this problem, medication compliance suddenly improved greatly. At follow-up, the patient was able to sit at 30° recline, primarily to accommodate her hip extension contracture, and with a reverse wedge seat and hardware adjustments could again use an upright manual or power wheelchair and return to school part-time.

In the present patient, the main presenting problems (see table) were accompanied by additional factors related to pain: active synovitis, renal stone formation, osteopenia, and neuropathic (complex regional pain) syndrome due to immobilization post-injury and self-immobilization. JRA is usually an "outpatient" disease; only extraordinary cases such as this one, with years of uncontrolled disease activity and severe complications of osteopenia and immobility, are referred for inpatient rehabilitation. Family noncompliance apparently stemmed from beliefs about disability, particularly inability to walk, and long-term prognosis of JRA as well as poor appreciation of control vs. lack of control of underlying disease activity. They did not in any way want their child to die when a real and immediate threat became apparent, and once the possibility of improvement rather than continued deterioration was clearly demonstrated, the family became completely compliant with treatment.

Clinical Pearls

1. Sometimes there is no substitute for a comprehensive, coordinated, expanded rehabilitation team effort—including the appropriate medical specialists—to unravel and solve complex and severe medical and functional problems. (Author's note: Even the insurance company that frequently balks at inpatient coverage paid for this stay in its entirety.)

2. When narcotic pain medication is ineffective, and pain with motion is extraordinary, consider neuropathic pain and try appropriate therapy.

3. Lesser, more realistic goals can still make an enormous difference in the life of a rehabilitation patient, both in quality and quantity.

REFERENCES

1. Allen G, Galer BS, Schwartz L: Epidemiology of complex regional pain syndrome: a retrospective chart review of 134 patients. Pain 80(3):539–44, 1999.
2. Bushnell TG, Cobo-Castro T: Complex regional pain syndrome: becoming more or less complex? Man Ther 4(4):221–228, 1999.
3. Harden RN, Cole P: New developments in rehabilitation of neuropathic pain syndromes. Neurol Clin 16(4):937–950, 1998.
4. Henderson CJ, Specker BL, Sierra RI, Campaigne BN, Lovell DJ: Total-body bone mineral content in non-corticosteroid-treated postpubertal females with juvenile rheumatoid arthritis: frequency of osteopenia and contributing factors. Arthritis Rheum 43(3):531–540, 2000.
5. Moriwaki K, Yuge O, Tanaka H, et al: Neuropathic pain and prolonged regional inflammation as two distinct symptomatological components in complex regional pain syndrome with patchy osteoporosis—a pilot study. Pain 72(1-2):277–82, 1997.
6. Rabinovich CE: Bone mineral status in juvenile rheumatoid arthritis. J Rheumatol 27 Suppl 58:34–37, 2000.

PATIENT 59

A 79-year-old man with chronic low back pain

A 79-year-old man presents with a 4-month history of low back pain and fever of unknown origin. Prior to developing back pain he was quite active, walking three miles a day. He was evaluated at the local hospital and found to have pneumonia on chest x-ray and degenerative disc disease of the lumbar spine on lumbosacral spine x-rays. He was treated with intravenous antibiotics and discharged to home. Unfortunately, he continued to decline over the next several months, with lower extremity weakness and bowel and bladder incontinence developing. He is now readmitted to the hospital for further work-up.

Physical Examination: Temperature 101°, pulse 98, respiration 18, blood pressure 160/72. HEENT: normal. Chest: clear. Cardiac: normal. Abdomen: distended but nontender, with hypoactive bowel sounds. Musculoskeletal: normal peripheral joints; back pain with any movement and tender to palpation over upper lumbar spine. Extremities: no swelling or edema noted in feet; normal bilateral pedal pulses. Neurologic: intact but mildly impaired sensation to touch and pinprick of bilateral lower extremities; hyperreflexic muscle stretch reflexes in bilateral lower extremities at knees and ankles, with 10 beats of ankle clonus; manual muscle test limited secondary to back pain, but at least antigravity strength at hips and knees and 4/5 strength with ankle dorsiflexion and plantarflexion. Skin: blanchable redness over bilateral heels. Genitourinary: Foley catheter in place, with straw-colored urine in drainage bag.

Laboratory Findings: WBC 17,000/µl , hct 35.7%; platelets 199,000/µl. Prothrombin time 12.8 seconds; partial thromboplastin time 32 seconds. Electrolytes, BUN, creatinine: normal. Chest x-ray: no active pulmonary disease, mildly enlarged heart. MRI of T-spine and L-spine: see figure.

Question: What is the cause of this patient's back pain?

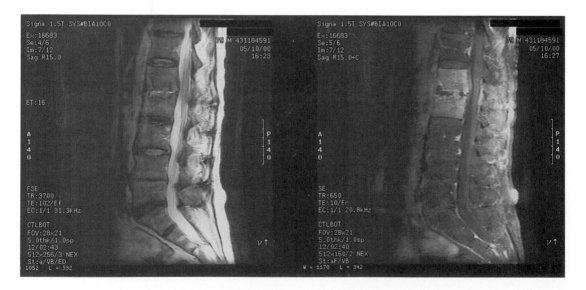

Diagnosis: Discitis secondary to methicillin-sensitive *Staphylococcus aureus*.

Discussion: Discitis is inflammation of the intervertebral disc secondary to infection or benign inflammation. It presents clinically as childhood discitis, adult disc space infection, postsurgical disc space infection, or direct infection (trauma) to the intervertebral disc. The disc has a vascular supply; thus it can become infected by the hematogenous route (however, some argue that the vascular supply is absent in the adult), adjacent osteomyelitis, or direct inoculation. The persistence of back pain, muscle spasm, difficulty walking, and an elevated erythrocyte sedimentation rate 4–6 weeks after surgery is suggestive of disc space infection. The incidence after vertebral disc surgery is 1.0–2.8%; after discography it is 1% with single-needle technique and 0.5% with double-needle technique.

Childhood discitis is disc inflammation that presents as clinically severe back pain with radiological evidence of disc space narrowing and involvement of adjacent vertebral end plates. The inflammation is usually benign and tends to involve only a single intervertebral disc. Clinical recovery occurs rapidly over 72 hours. Complete or partial restoration of disk height is seen in most children within 6 weeks to 1 year. Immobilization is only used if there is not a rapid and dramatic response. Some clinicians use immobilization alone, and only start antibiotics if immobilization is ineffective. Primary discitis does occur in adults, but the course may not be benign and may not resolve spontaneously.

Discitis secondary to infection usually involves *S. aureus* and can be the result of direct infection or hematogenous spread. Management is similar to the treatment for osteomyelitis, and antibiotic treatment should be directed by the culture results and of 4- to 6-week duration. *Mycobacterium tuberculosis* can occur in any bone; however, common locations in adults are the vertebral bodies of the thoracic spine, where destruction of the vertebral body and the disk may be the result. Prolonged chemotherapy and possible surgery is needed for an infection with *M. tuberculosis*.

In the present patient, the MRI revealed multiple level degenerative disc disease of the lumbar spine, worse at L4–5. Most significant, though, was the discitis at L1–2 with extension into the L1 and L2 vertebral bodies. The patient underwent a CT-guided biopsy and drainage of the L1–2 disc. Cultures were positive for methicillin-sensitive S. aureus. He was treated with immobilization via a thoracolumbosacral orthosis and was started on a 6-week course of intravenous Ancef, 1 g every 8 hours. His back pain slowly resolved, and he regained full strength in his legs. Spasticity also resolved. He did not develop any signs of neurogenic bowel or bladder.

Clinical Pearls

1. Low back pain and fever are red flags for possible infection in the low back, especially after an invasive procedure to the spine.
2. Treatment with antibiotics is similar to the treatment course for osteomyelitis and should be directed by culture results to be successful.
3. Primary discitis in childhood is usually benign and resolves spontaneously, but in adults the course is more variable and may not be benign.

REFERENCES
1. Green NE: Bone and joint infections in children. In Weinstein SL, Buckwalter JA (eds): Turek's Orthopaedics: Principles and Their Application, 5th ed. Philadelphia, JB Lippincott, 1994.
2. Mader JT, Calhoun J: Osteomyelitis. In Mandell GL (ed): Principles of Practice of Infectious Disease, 5th ed. Philadelphia, Churchill Livingstone, 2000.
3. Wood GW II: Infections of the spine. In Canale ST (ed): Campbell's Operative Orthopaedics. New York, Mosby, 1998, pp 3102–3103.

PATIENT 60

A 69-year-old woman with thoracolumbar pain occurring after shoulder surgery

A 69-year-old woman is referred with progressively increasing thoracolumbar pain. Insidious onset occurred 4 months ago while she was hospitalized for a total shoulder replacement. After surgery she developed a low-grade fever which was treated with oral antibiotics for 2 weeks. She was discharged with residual back pain. An MRI of the lumbar spine revealed severe spinal stenosis at L3-L4/L4-L5. She failed to respond to physical therapy and chiropractic manipulation. All of the treatment received was primarily for her low back. Her past medical history is noncontributory, with no risk factors for HIV infection or other predisposing factors such as diabetes mellitus, IV drug abuse, or chronic alcoholism.

Physical Examination: General: acute distress due to back pain; all movements slow and guarded. Vital signs: normal. Musculoskeletal: very tender area of muscle spasms in mid-thoracic and upper lumbar region; loss of all spinal movements. Neurologic: straight leg raise negative bilaterally; normal stretch reflexes and sensation.

Laboratory Findings: WBC: mildly elevated. Serum chemistries: normal. ESR: 66 mm/hr (elevated). Serum protein electrophoresis: alpha II elevation consistent with inflammatory process. HIV: negative. Blood cultures: negative. Electrodiagnostic study: acute and severe denervation in lower thoracic paraspinal muscles; no evidence of peripheral involvement. Radiographs of thoracic spine: active discitis at T8-T9; osteomyelitis and bone destruction.

Questions: Which imaging studies will help confirm a diagnosis? What is the organism responsible for this condition? What was the source of the infection?

Answers: Magnetic resonance imaging can confirm a diagnosis. *Candida tropicalis* is responsible, and surgical instrumentation may have been the source.

Discussion: Fungal spondylodiscitis is an uncommon condition. However, its incidence appears to be on the rise, probably related to the increased number of immunocompromised patients and intravenous drug abusers. This condition usually occurs through hematogenous spread from infected foci in the body or by direct extension from instrumentation or surgery.

Disc space infection with associated vertebral osteomyelitis (spondylodiscitis) is an inflammatory process, which seems to have a predilection for the lumbar region. However, the thoracic region can be involved almost as commonly. To make a diagnosis, the condition must be suspected: note that fever and other constitutional symptoms are often absent, and x-ray changes may not be present for weeks. The **ESR** is invariably elevated and should be checked in any patient whose course is prolonged or otherwise atypical, or who is a member of a high-risk group (i.e., those who have had recent pelvic infection or back surgery, IV drug abusers, children and adolescents with back pain). Early diagnosis is imperative to prevent or minimize serious complications, which could include permanent paralysis.

Vertebral osteomyelitis is usually secondary to *Staphylococcus aureus* or, in needle users, to gram-negative organisms. Candida osteomyelitis is a rare entity. A review of the literature done in 1987 revealed only 32 case reports of Candida osteomyelitis in adults. However, as the incidence of candidiasis continues to increase in immunocompromised patients, this condition will be seen more frequently.

When Candida involves the spine, it is usually centered around the intervertebral disc space, with narrowing of the disc cartilage causing destruction and lysis of the vertebral plates and underlying vertebral bone. This condition is typically **insidious** in nature. It is uncommon to have associated symptoms such as low-grade fever or chills. The most useful clinical finding to identify spondylodiscitis is to evoke **point tenderness** over the affected area, with paravertebral tenderness. Common predisposing factors associated with this condition include: diabetes mellitus, extreme age, IV drug abuse, intravenous access, discography, infective endocarditis, urinary tract infections, chronic alcoholism, and immunodepressive states.

Diagnosis is confirmed using radiographic or imaging studies. Normally, radiographic changes in vertebral osteomyelitis are present 2–8 weeks after the onset. The appearance of **vertebral osteomyelitis on MRI** is characteristic. MRI is more accurate and sensitive than radioisotope, bone scan, or CT scan for early recognition and localization of infectious disease in patients suspected of having this condition. This is also an excellent way of demonstrating the presence of any epidural or paraspinal extension of the infection. Intravenous antibiotics in combination with anterior debridement and spinal fusion gives good, early, and long-term results, with rapid recovery and low morbidity and mortality.

The present patient represents an unusual case of spondylodiscitis due to Candida with no predisposing factors. An MRI of her thoracic spine confirmed the presence of osteomyelitis, with bone destruction and compromise of the spinal cord (see figure). She was admitted to the hospital where she underwent a vertebrectomy, debridement, and fusion. Cultures from the spine were reported as positive for fungi, which eventually grew out as *Candida tropicalis*. The patient was started on intravenous amphotericin B and vancomycin. After 12 weeks of therapy she was much improved and was discharged home in a brace. This unusual case reaffirms the necessity of a careful physical examination and a high index of suspicion to obtain an early and accurate diagnosis.

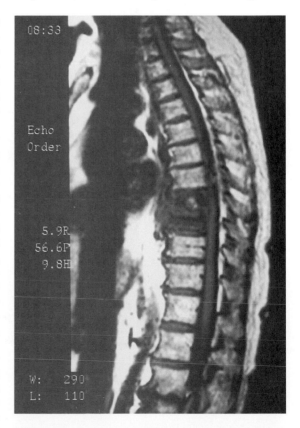

MRI saggital T1-weighted view revealing active discitis at T8-T9.

Clinical Pearls

1. Disc space infection with vertebral osteomyelitis (spondylodiscitis) due to fungus infection is an uncommon condition.
2. The most useful clinical finding is point tenderness over the affected area.
3. Spondylodiscitis must be suspected in patients with uncharacteristically severe, localized back pain.
4. The sedimentation rate in spondylodiscitis is invariably elevated.
5. Radiologic imaging confirms the diagnosis, and MRI is the procedure of choice.

REFERENCES

1. Derkinderen P, Bruneel F, Bouchaud O, et al: Spondylodiscitis and epidural abscess due to candida albicans. Eur Spine J 9(1):72–74, 2000.
2. Lifeso RM: Pyogenic Spinal Sepsis in Adults. Spine 15:1265–1271, 1990.
3. Malowski SK, Lukowski S: Pyogenic Infection of the Spine. Clin Orthop Rel Research 272:58–66,1991.
4. Smith A, Blaser S: Infections and Inflammatory Processes of the Spine. Radiol Clin North Am 29(4):809–827, 1991.
5. Wirtz DC, Genius I, Wildberger JE: Diagnostic and therapeutic management of lumbar and thoracic spondylodiscitis—An evaluation of 59 cases. Arch Orthop Trauma Surg 12(5–6):245–251, 2000.

PATIENT 61

A 28-year-old woman with a history of leg weakness and falls

A 28-year-old woman complains of a history of foot and ankle pain and frequent falls that have increased over the last decade. The patient states that she has difficulty wearing high-heeled shoes and is self-conscious about the clawed appearance of her toes. She denies any upper extremity weakness. Upon questioning, she remembers that her grandmother, who is now deceased, had similar foot characteristics. The patient also reports a history of foot ulcerations on the sole of her foot that tend to recur frequently.

Physical Examination: General: thin; no acute distress; alert and oriented. Musculoskeletal: bilateral gastrocnemius and extensor digitorum brevis atrophy bilaterally; clawed toes bilaterally; flexible pes cavus deformity, which flattens to pes planus deformity with mild equinovarus in stance; 5/5 strength in hip flexors, hip extensors, knee flexors, and knee extensors bilaterally; 3/5 strength in bilateral dorsiflexors and plantar flexors. Gait: reciprocal, with normal stride lengths; occasional catching of forefoot on floor. Neurologic: decreased proprioception in lower extremities; pinprick and soft touch sensation intact; reflexes 1+ patella tendon, but absent at Achilles.

Laboratory Findings: CBC normal. ESR, rheumatoid factor, ANA: negative. X-ray of bilateral feet (*see figure*): pes cavus deformity of arch; no fractures or osteoporosis. Electrodiagnostic studies: nerve conduction velocities of bilateral tibial nerves—left 32 m/s, right 33 m/s; electromyography of left and right gastrocnemius—2+ fibrillations, 2+ positive sharp waves.

Question: What is the most likely diagnosis of this patient's apparent symmetrical lower extremity weakness?

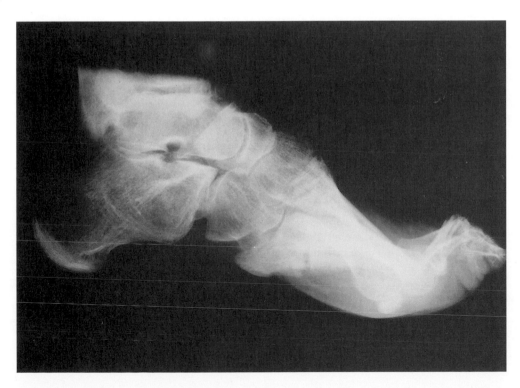

Answer: Charcot-Marie-Tooth disease (hereditary motor sensory neuropathy).

Discussion: Charcot-Marie-Tooth (CMT) is the most common peripheral neuropathic disorder seen in clinical practice today. It was described in the late 1800s by Charcot-Marie, and separately by Tooth. Due to ongoing research, this disease is now characterized as a genetically heterogeneous disorder referred to as **hereditary motor sensory neuropathy** (HMSN). It is characterized by variable penetrance with multiple forms, most of which can be delineated through careful electrodiagnostic testing and nerve and muscle biopsy. Currently, there are seven types of HMSN; however, this discussion focuses on HMSN 1 and HMSN 2.

HMSN 1 is the most common form of this peripheral neuropathy and accounts for approximately 61% of all cases (including the present patient). This form is also known as hypertrophic CMT due to an association of enlarged nerves and prominent onion bulb formation on nerve biopsy. History usually includes complaints of falling and gait abnormalities. Foot and ankle deformities usually include pes cavus, claw toes, equinovarus of the forefoot, and Achilles tendon contractures.

Electrodiagnosis, including EMG and nerve conduction studies, are a critical part of diagnosing separate forms of HMSN. Criteria for diagnosis for HMSN1 include nerve conduction velocities less than 40 meters per second with severely reduced compound motor action potentials. EMG findings include decreased recruitment increased amplitude of motor unit action potentials, polyphasia, positive sharp waves, and fibrillations. Nerve conduction studies also show decreased or absent sensory nerve action potentials amplitude and prolonged latencies. HMSN 1 is therefore thought to be a uniform, segmental, demyelinating process.

In contrast, **HMSN 2**, also known as the neuronal form of CMT, typically presents in older patients, usually in their second to fourth decade. The mode of inheritance is thought to be autosomal dominant; however, a recessive form has been reported. Plantar flexor weakness is more often seen in HMSN 2, while HMSN 1 can have more prominent involvement of the upper extremities.

Electrodiagnostic criteria for HMSN 2 include nerve conduction velocities never below 60% of normal, latencies only mildly prolonged, and normal amplitude and wave form in the compound motor action potential. Electrodiagnostic studies show no evidence of segmental demyelination, but do demonstrate axonal degeneration. Nerve biopsy differs as there are no onion bulb formations. Autopsies have revealed a degeneration in the anterior horn cells in the lumbosacral region in the HMSN 2 form.

Two theories exist on the pathogenesis of HMSN 1 and HMSN 2. Some authors feel that the defect primarily lies in the axon itself, while others feel that demyelination is due to the primary defect in the myelin or Schwann cells.

Lower extremity deformities are common in CMT. They are believed to result from a muscular imbalance between the intrinsic muscles of the foot and extrinsic muscles of the leg. Patients complain of foot pain, ulcers, and ill-fitting shoes. Hammer toes and pes cavus are often seen. Treatment of these deformities should begin early, with extensive evaluation by rehabilitation professionals. Patients are felt to benefit from early therapeutic exercise, orthotics, and custom shoe modification. Orthotic management may include plastic ankle-foot orthosis (AFO) to offset foot drop; however, due to sensory changes, metal double-upright AFOs attached to the shoe may be more appropriate.

Clinical Pearls

1. Charcot-Marie-Tooth disease, also called hereditary motor sensory neuropathy, is a common form of a peripheral neuropathy.
2. Electrodiagnostic studies are key to the diagnosis of CMT.
3. Rehabilitation services including therapeutic exercise, orthotic management, and shoe modification should be initiated early to improve functional outcomes.

REFERENCE
Njegovan ME, Leonard EI, Joseph FB: Rehabilitation medicine approach to Charcot-Marie-Tooth disease. Clin Podiatr Med Surg 14(1):99–116, 1997.

PATIENT 62

A 76-year-old man with hip and thigh pain after a fall

A 76-year-old man and his wife of 51 years were out walking on a nature trail when he tripped over a fallen branch, landing directly on his right side. He had a lot of pain in his right hip and proximal thigh, as well as his groin. He attempted to stand, but was unable due to the severity of the pain. His wife called an ambulance, and he was taken to a local emergency department. The couple live a very active life, enjoying a number of hobbies and recreational activities. He is in good health except for mild hypertension and osteoarthritis.

Physical Examination: Blood pressure 162/95, pulse 110, respirations 22, temperature 99°. Extremities: point tenderness in right proximal lateral femur and anterior thigh; no obvious deformity; much swelling and hematoma at region of tenderness; pulses palpable and symmetric in distal lower extremities. Neurologic: intact in lower extremities. Musculoskeletal: pain in right hip and proximal femur with any passive range of motion. Cardiac: increased rate, normal rhythm. Chest: clear. Abdomen: benign.

Laboratory Findings: X-ray of hip (*see figure*): partially displaced femoral neck fracture; moderate osteoarthritis.

Course: The patient is evaluated and stabilized by the orthopedic surgeon on call. His extremity is placed in slight hip flexion and external rotation to minimize stresses on the joint, and he is medically cleared for a right total hip replacement, which takes place later that evening. Cemented femoral and acetabular components are placed via posterior approach.

Question: What are the typical postoperative hip precautions, including weight-bearing status, for this patient?

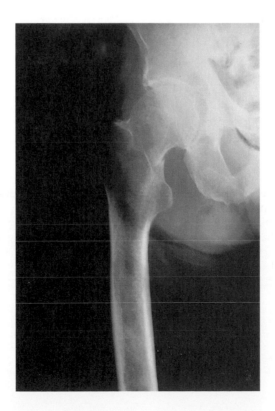

Answer: Avoid the following: hip flexion beyond 90 degrees, hip adduction past midline, hip internal rotation, and side lying without abductor pillow. Full weight-bearing as tolerated using a walker is allowed as soon as the day after surgery.

Discussion: The incidence of hip fractures has increased dramatically as a result of our expanding elderly population; 95% of hip fractures occur in people aged 50 years or older. The primary goals in performing a total hip replacement after a hip fracture or in the presence of severe osteoarthritis are to restore function and minimize morbidity. **Cemented prostheses**, introduced in 1961, are the better choice for the elderly for two main reasons: (1) the uncemented, porous implant is a less stable prosthesis for aged individuals, and (2) the patient receiving the uncemented component must be non-weight-bearing or limited weight-bearing. Both of these factors greatly increase the risks for morbidity and mortality. Uncemented endoprostheses are more commonly used in younger individuals who have a greater bone density and are better able to effectively create bony ingrowth into the porous surface.

Certain patients are not surgical candidates due to various medical problems. Note that the mortality rate following a hip fracture is significantly higher in people who are treated nonsurgically. Mortality in nonsurgical patients is primarily a result of the complications of immobility, including pneumonia and pulmonary embolism. Common forms of morbidity include pressure sores, deep venous thrombosis, flexion contractures, deconditioning, and emotional decline.

The present patient recovered well from his surgery. While open reduction with internal fixation would normally be a reasonable surgical choice for his type of fracture, the total hip replacement was ideal for him in light of his underlying acetabular osteoarthritis. His rehabilitation spanned 6 weeks, and consisted of both physical therapy and occupational therapy. He was fully weight-bearing using a walker by the second postoperative day. X-rays were taken at 4, 6, and 12 weeks to ensure that the prosthesis was intact, and warfarin was prescribed for 6 weeks as prophylaxis against deep vein thrombosis.

The first week consisted primarily of reinforcement of hip precautions (outlined above), lower extremity exercises, range of motion, transfer training, use of assistive devices, training in activities of daily living, and pulmonary toilet. Adhering to hip precautions is especially vital for this patient because total hip replacement via the posterior approach has a higher incidence of postoperative dislocation compared with the anterior and lateral approaches.

The second week consisted of advancing his exercise program and distance walking as well as practicing climbing stairs and doing a car transfer. The rest of his rehabilitation took place on an outpatient basis. His home equipment consisted of an abductor pillow, a raised toilet seat, a reacher, and bathroom grab bars. During the third week he advanced to a cane and received home health physical therapy once a day for 1 week. During weeks 4-6, he continued with his home exercises and increased his strength and endurance.

Clinical Pearls

1. Of patients with hip fracture, 95% are 50 years of age or older.

2. The incidence of hip fractures has markedly increased owing to our increasing elderly population.

3. Due to complications from immobility, the mortality rate is much higher in seniors with hip fractures that are treated conservatively, compared with those that are treated surgically.

4. People with cemented total hip replacements are cleared to fully bear weight as tolerated as early as 1 day following surgery.

5. Adhering to total hip precautions is especially vital for people who underwent a posterior surgical approach, because this approach has a higher incidence of postoperative dislocation compared to lateral or anterior approaches.

REFERENCES

1. Brander VA, Hinderer SR, Alpiner N, Oh TH: Limb disorders. Arch Phys Med Rehabil 76(5-suppl):S47–56, 1995.
2. Cifu DX, Burnett D, McGowan JP: Rehabilitation after hip fracture. In Grabois M, Garrison SJ, Hart KA, Lehmkuhl LD (eds): Physical Medicine and Rehabilitation: The Complete Approach. Malden, MA, Blackwell Science, 2000, pp 1534–1550.
3. Genova A: Hip Pain. A Lecture at The West Los Angeles VA Medical Center, 1996.
4. National Institutes of Health Consensus Development Conference: Total Hip Replacement. Baltimore, MD, September 12–14, 1994.

PATIENT 63

A 72-year-old man having difficulty walking and frequent falls

A 72-year-old man has been experiencing difficulty walking and frequent falls for the past month. He falls about twice a week because he trips over his left toes. He also complains of low back pain for the past month.

Physical Examination: General: ambulates with steppage gait on left. Musculoskeletal: weakness in dorsiflexion of left foot. Neurologic: sensation intact to light touch in lower extremities, except decreased in left first web space; reflexes symmetrically decreased.

Laboratory Findings: See results of nerve conduction and EMG studies below.

Question: Why is this man falling?

Nerve Conduction Study

Nerve	Site	Latency	CV	Amplitude
L deep peroneal (m)	Ankle-EDB	5.2 msec		0.9 mV
	FH-ankle		36 m/s	0.5 mV
	Pop fossa-FH		48 m/s	0.4 mV
L deep peroneal (m)	FH-tib ant	4.0 msec		3.0 mV
	Pop fossa-FH		42 m/s	2.6 mV
L tibial (m)	Ankle-AH	4.2 msec		4.0 mV
	Pop fossa-ankle		42 m/s	3.0 mV
L sural (s)	Mid-calf-ankle	3.9 msec	36 m/s	10 µV
R deep peroneal (m)	Ankle-EDB	3.8 msec		4.0 mV
	FH-ankle		46 m/s	3.6 mV
	Pop fossa-FH		43 m/s	3.4 mV
R sural (s)	Mid-calf-ankle	3.9 msec	36 m/s	15 µV

(m) = motor, (s) = sensory, CV = conduction velocity, EDB = extensor digitorum brevis, FH = fibular head, AH = abductor hallucis

EMG Study

Muscle	Insertional Activity	MUAP Morphology	MUAP Recruitment
L VMO	Normal	Normal	Normal
L anterior tibialis	2+ fibs/PSW	50% polyphasics	Mildly decreased
L EHL	2+ fibs/PSW	50% polyphasics	Mildly decreased
L peroneus longus	Occas. fib	Normal	Normal
L medial gastroc	Normal	Normal	Normal
L biceps femoris-short head	Normal	Normal	Normal
L gluteus medius	Normal	Normal	Normal
L lumbar paraspinals	Normal	—	—

VMO = vastus medialis obliquus, PSW = positive sharp waves, EHL = extensor hallucis longus, MUAP = motor unit action potential, fibs = fibrillation potentials

Diagnosis: Left peroneal neuropathy at the fibular head

Discussion: The differential diagnosis of a foot drop includes mononeuropathies of the deep peroneal, common peroneal, and/or sciatic nerves, lumbosacral plexopathy, L5 radiculopathy, motor neuron disease, and cerebral lesions. In this case, the clinical exam results suggest a peroneal nerve lesion, and the electrodiagnostic test confirms this diagnosis.

The common peroneal nerve is formed from the lateral portion of the sciatic nerve and receives innervation from the L4 to S2 nerve roots. As it courses distally, it gives off at about the mid-thigh a branch to the short head of the biceps femoris. Typically, the sciatic nerve divides into the tibial and common peroneal nerves just proximal to the popliteal fossa. Both the common peroneal and tibial nerves contribute fibers to the sural nerve, and the common peroneal gives off a branch to the lateral cutaneous nerve of the thigh. The common peroneal nerve then crosses the lateral gastrocnemius muscle and becomes superficial as it courses distal to the fibular head.

Typically, the common peroneal nerve divides into the superficial and deep branches near the fibular head. The deep peroneal nerve innervates the muscles in the anterior compartment of the leg and the extensor digitorum brevis and extensor hallicus brevis. It provides sensory fibers to the **first web space**. The superficial peroneal nerve innervates the peroneous longus and brevis of the lateral compartment and provides sensory fibers to the dorsum of the foot. Due to the intraneural topography of the nerve fibers, the superficial peroneal nerve tends to be relatively spared with injuries at the fibular head.

For suspected peroneal nerve injuries, the following studies are recommended: nerve conduction studies of the deep peroneal nerves (with recording electrodes over the extensor digitorum brevis and tibialis anterior muscles) and the superficial peroneal sensory nerves; needle examination of two deep peroneal muscles, one superficial peroneal muscle, the biceps femoris-short head, another L5 innervated muscle (i.e., tibialis posterior, glutei muscles, or tensor fascia lata), and the lumbar paraspinals. In this author's experience, deep peroneal nerve conductions are not typically performed with the recording electrodes over the tibialis anterior unless the EDB is atrophied and CMAP amplitude recorded over the EDB is very reduced in size (as was the case in the present patient).

To distinguish between a radiculopathy and a peripheral nerve lesion, the examiner should find abnormalities on EMG needle exam in two muscles innervated by the same peripheral nerve, but different nerve roots. EMG exam of muscles innervated by the same nerve root but a different peripheral nerve should be normal. The paraspinal muscle should also be normal.

Clinical Pearls

1. The biceps femoris-short head is the only muscle proximal to the knee that is innervated by the peroneal nerve.

2. The superficial peroneal nerve is relatively spared in peroneal lesions at the fibular head.

3. Paraspinal needle exam should be normal if the foot drop is due to a peroneal nerve lesion or lumbosacral plexopathy.

REFERENCE

1. Esselman PC, Tomski MA, Robinson LR, et al: Selective deep peroneal nerve injury associated with arthroscopic knee surgery. Muscle Nerve 16:1188–1192, 1993.
2. Katirji B: Peroneal neuropathy. Neurol Clinics 17:567–591, 1999.
3. Levin KH, Stevens JC, Daube JR: Superficial peroneal nerve conduction studies for electrodiagnostic diagnosis. Muscle Nerve 9:322–326, 1986.
4. Miller RG: AAEM Minimongraph # 28: Injury to peripheral motor nerves. Muscle Nerve 10:698–710, 1987.
5. Wilbourn AJ: AAEM Case Report # 12: Common peroneal mononeuropathy at the fibular head. Muscle Nerve 9:825–836, 1986.

PATIENT 64

A 61-year-old man with sudden onset of dysphagia and ataxia

A 61-year-old man with a history of hypertension experienced sudden dizziness, nausea, and vomiting. He later noted difficulty swallowing and poor balance with a tendency to fall to the left. His family mentions that his voice has developed a nasal quality. He has not had any loss of consciousness or seizure.

Physical Examination: Blood pressure 170/80, pulse 92, respiration 18, temperature 97.8°. General: alert; not in acute distress; Dobhoff nasogastric feeding tube in place. Neurologic: oriented to person, place, and time; no agitation; speech hypophonic, but intelligible; cranial nerves grossly intact from II–XII; sensation diminished to pain and temperature on left face and right upper and lower extremities. Musculoskeletal: strength $4^+/5$–$5/5$ in all extremities; muscle stretch reflexes +2; dysmetria in right upper extremity. Gait: wide-based, inability to perform tandem walking, requiring minimal to contact-guard assistance for balance.

Laboratory Findings: Modified barium swallow study: mild slowing in oral phase; aspiration of thin liquids in pharyngeal phase.

Question: In what part of the brain is the lesion that accounts for these findings?

Diagnosis: Right lateral medulla

Discussion: Adolf Wallenberg first described the lateral medullary syndrome in 1895; hence, it is also known as Wallenberg syndrome. It is almost always due to an ischemic infarct in a portion of the medulla oblongata, lying posterior to the inferior olivary nucleus (see figure). The syndrome had traditionally been attributed to occlusion of the posterior inferior cerebellar artery (PICA syndrome), but studies have shown that in 80% of patients, the vertebral artery is the one occluded.

Classically, the manifestations are the following (with the corresponding anatomic site involved):

1. *Contralateral* impairment of pain and temperature on half of the body (spinothalamic tract)

2. Pain, numbness, impaired sensation over the the *ipsilateral* half of the face (descending tract and nucleus of the fifth cranial nerve)

3. *Ipsilateral* Horner's syndrome, with miosis, ptosis, and anhidrosis (descending sympathetic tract)

4. Nystagmus, vertigo, nausea, and/or vomiting (vestibular nuclei)

5. Hoarseness, dysphagia, diminished gag reflex, ipsilateral paralysis of the palate and vocal cord (issuing fibers of the ninth and tenth cranial nerves)

6. *Ipsilateral* ataxia of limbs, falling to ipsilateral side (olivocerebellar, and/or spinocerebellar fibers)

7. Loss of taste (nucleus and tractus solitarius)

8. Rarely, numbness of the *ipsilateral* limbs (nuclei cuneatus and gracilis).

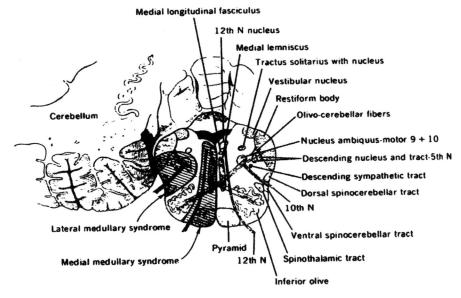

From Adams RD, Victor M (eds): Principles of Neurology, 6th ed. New York, McGraw-Hill, 1997; with permission.

Clinical Pearls

1. Ischemic infarction of the lateral medulla has traditionally been attributed to occlusion of the posterior inferior cerebellar artery, but in 8 out of 10 cases, the vertebral artery is the one involved.

2. The clinical presentation of Wallenberg syndrome is variable and depends on the anatomic areas affected.

REFERENCES

1. Adams RD, Victor M (eds): Principles of Neurology, 6th ed. New York, McGgraw-Hill, 1997.
2. Kirsteins AE, Black-Schaffer RM, Harvey RL: Stroke rehabilitation. 3. Rehabilitation management. Arch Phys Med Rehabil 80:S17–S20, 1999.

PATIENT 65

A 6-year-old boy with delayed development and suspected cerebral palsy

A 6-year-old boy is brought to an outreach clinic with concerns about possible cerebral palsy and need for therapy and orthotic management. He was born at 36 weeks gestation in a regular, vaginal delivery and weighed 5 pounds. Some lung problems were initially present, but only a 3-day hospital stay was required. He had one episode of pneumonia at age 3. He takes supplemental iron, but no other medications. Development was reportedly very slow: he rolled over at 9 months, sat at age 2, pulled to stand shortly after, and walked at age 3. He toe walks intermittently now, but he still can't run and falls frequently. The patient's mother states that he is to repeat kindergarten this year. He needs help with dressing.

A recent vision test was normal; he may not have had a hearing test, as he usually "talks your ear off." He has a healthy and typically developing full sibling who is 1 year older, as well as two half-siblings, both healthy. There is no family history of muscle disease. Neuroimaging and blood work have not been performed. Orthotics were once prescribed, but he did not get them and has no current formal therapy.

Physical Examination: HEENT: remarkable only for slight scarring of both tympanic membranes; no infections; no adenopathy. Chest: clear. Cardiac: good sinus arrhythmia and split S2 (normal.) Musculoskeletal: uses hands to brace himself when getting up to stand; firm, large calf muscles (subtle hypertrophy—see figure); heelcord ROM is just to neutral. Neurologic: equivocal Babinski reflexes and hypoactive to normal (1+) deep tendon reflexes. Gait: mildly affected, with excess lateral sway and lordosis; he does not try to do tandem or heel gaits when requested and demonstrated. Manual muscle test: patient cannot cooperate.

Questions: What is a more likely diagnosis than cerebral palsy? What should be checked to quickly confirm or refute the alternate diagnosis?

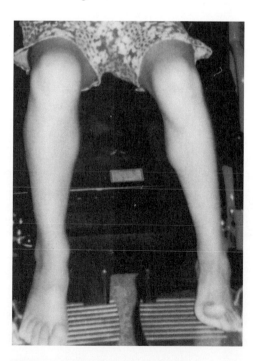

Diagnosis: Duchenne's muscular dystrophy. Check the creatine phosphokinase level.

Discussion: This patient's CPK level of 9754 IU/L is near the maximal recordable for this machine at a small rural hospital. The disorder is almost certainly Duchenne's muscular dystrophy (DMD); the CPK should be five digits, and in the absence of any history of physical findings of myositis or rhabdomyolsis, nothing else will produce this degree of elevation. DMD often presents this way, as nonspecific, seemingly global developmental delays, and is often managed as mild cerebral palsy in error in the early years. It may even present as "floppy baby syndrome" (hypotonia in infancy), which usually is then readily diagnosed because the high CPK is present from birth.

In hypotonia, the most important differential is weak versus not weak. Mild or no relative weakness indicates cerebral, metabolic, or other global pathologies. Definite weakness, determined by observation of antigravity functioning in children who cannot cooperate with manual muscle testing, suggest neuromuscular diseases (anterior horn cell, peripheral nerve, neuromuscular junction, or muscle pathology). Spinal cord disorders can present as hypotonia, but often with a sensory level. Children with all of these disorders occasionally come to physiatric attention bearing a diagnosis of "cerebral palsy."

Therapists unfamiliar with the biomechanics of a DMD gait may focus on toe-walking and mildly tight heel cords and recommend the orthotic management they would prescribe for a child with cerebral palsy—therapy that is unnecessary and unhelpful. **DNA analysis** for dystrophin is the next confirmatory step, and could offer valuable information about suitability for experimental treament; if a premature "stop codon," which halts transcription of the dystrophin protein, is found, gentamycin may be tried (experimental) to override this genetically. DNA analysis also aids in genetic evaluation of potential carriers—his mother and any close female relatives on her side.

Learning disabilities, particularly for math, and/or slightly lower IQs are not uncommon in DMD, but are by no means universal. Grade retention without psychoeducational testing is usually ill-advised if it is done in hopes of giving the student time to "catch up" physically with the other children; children with DMD become weaker. **Contracture prevention** is the focus of early physical therapy. Contracture can be mistaken for hypertonia, and children with dystrophinopathy can be at least mildly globally delayed. Providing information and educating our physical therapy colleagues, especially those less experienced or less familiar with neuromuscular disorders (some are experts in this area; others are unfamiliar) about the differences in presentation and management differences is usually well received. Despite side effects, early **steroid treament** also holds promise for longer-term preservation of muscle strength.

It is important to communicate to parents that this diagnosis is bad news, and that DMD will cause progressive weakness and disability. However, the discussion should be tempered with the information that a lifespan into the 30s, rather than the teens, is possible with good care and modern respiratory supports. Be sure to convey the realistic possiblity that the child will indeed live into adulthood, and therefore should be prepared for adulthood, rather than treated as terminally ill. Too often a sense of futility and imminent fatality is conveyed, and this is no longer appropriate or accurate.

Clinical Pearls

1. Cerebral palsy is sometimes referred to as a "wastebasket diagnosis," but it really isn't: despite multiple etiologies and a wide variety of presentations, it does have a specific definition (see Pearl no. 2).

2. Cerebral palsy is a motor disorder due to nonprogressive brain pathology with onset in the early developmental period. Not all children with motor delays have cerebral palsy.

3. In hypotonia, the most important differential is weak vs. not weak.

4. Contracture can be mistaken for hypertonia, and children with dystrophinopathy can be at least mildly globally delayed.

REFERENCES
1. The Muscular Dystrophy Association: Journey of Love: A Parent's Guide to Duchenne Muscular Dystrophy. Tucson, AZ, MDA, 1998 (write to 3300 East Sunrise Drive, zip code 85718).
2. Talkop UA, Klaassen T, Piirsoo A, et al: Duchenne and Becker muscular dystrophies: An Estonian experience. Brain Dev 21(4):244–247, 1999.
3. Warren, Horan, Stefans: Breathe easy: Options for respiratory care. Available at http://mdausa.org/publications/breathe/index.html

PATIENT 66

A 57-year-old man with acute paraparesis after an elective cholecystectomy

A 57-year-old man first noted bilateral lower extremity weakness after an elective laparoscopic cholycystectomy. When he awoke from general anesthesia his legs would not work well, but over the next 2–3 hours he regained some strength and was discharged to home with a follow-up scheduled with a local neurologist. His main complaint when he saw the neurologist was neck, back, and bilateral leg pain. He reported no bowel or bladder incontinence. He had an 8-year history of chronic low back pain after a work-related injury and was disabled due to low back pain. A nerve conduction study revealed mild left median nerve slowing and mild slowing of right tibial and peroneal nerve conduction. Myofascial strain and degenerative disc disease were conjectured, but the patient was scheduled for an MRI to rule out spine pathology. However, he did not keep the appointment, and the MRI was not obtained. A week later he developed paraplegia and started having trouble with bowel and bladder incontinence. He now presents in your office, referred by the state spinal cord case manager because of paraplegia and a sacral pressure ulcer. He is in a wheelchair and unable to move either lower extremity. He is very angry and talks of suing the physician who did the surgery and caused his paraplegia.

Physical Examination: Temperature 97.8°, pulse 82, respiration 14, blood pressure 110/74. HEENT: normal. Chest: clear. Cardiac: normal. Abdomen: nontender, with normal active bowel sounds. Musculoskeletal: back pain with any movement and point tenderness to palpation over mid thoracic spine. Neurologic: hyperreflexic muscle stretch reflexes with flexor spasms of bilateral lower extremities on minimal stimulation; 5/5 strength in bilateral upper extremities, 0/5 strength in bilateral lower extremities. Skin: large, stage three, sacral pressure ulcer with foul odor and a large amount of necrotic tissue.

Laboratory Findings: WBC 30,400/µl, hct 37.3 %, platelets 342,000 /µl. BUN 13 mg/dl, creatinine 0.6 mg/dl, albumin 2.4 g/dl. Chest x-ray: 8-cm mass in right hilar region; 2-cm mass in left mid lung field with left hilar lymphadenopathy (see figure).

Question: What is the cause of this patient's back pain and paraparesis?

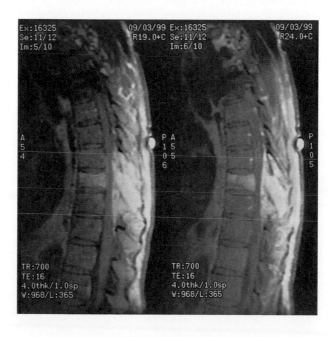

Diagnosis: Metastatic spinal tumor at T8 vertebral body.

Discussion: Spinal cord tumors may be *primary* or *metastatic*. They are classified as *extradural* or *intradural*, and the intradural tumors can be further subdivided into *intramedullary* or *extramedullary*. The majority of extradural lesions are neoplastic, arising from metastasis of the adjacent spinal column. **Neoplasms** originating in the lung, prostate, and breast are common; however, virtually every malignant tumor has been reported to cause metastatic epidural compression.

The initial symptom in epidural compression is usually local back pain, often worse in the recumbent position, and exacerbated by coughing, sneezing, or straining. Pain and local tenderness often proceed neurologic symptoms by several days to several weeks. The neurologic symptoms begin with progressive weakness and sensory loss and progress to paraparesis and a distinct sensory level. MRI is the optimal way to demonstrate cord compression and the nature of the pathology.

Extradural lesions in the thoracic region are typically metastatic in origin. The differential diagnosis of tumors in the thoracic region is difficult because of the lack of involvement of limbs early on in the disease process. It may be assumed that patients with T2–T6 lesions are suffering from angina or mediastinal pain. In individuals with T6–10 lesions, it is is not uncommon to have referred pain to the gallbladder, as was the case with the present patient. Since the two disease processes are not mutually exclusive, a surgeon can remove a diseased gallbladder only to have the patient continue to complain of pain because of the spinal cord tumor. Finally, a tumor below T10 can cause signs and symptoms referred to the inguinal, flank, and posterior subcostal regions—suggestive of, for example, renal colic or appendicitis.

Intradural, extramedullary tumors are less frequent and evolve more slowly clinically. Meningiomas and neurofibromas are most common. Symptoms usually begin with radicular sensory changes and an asymmetric spinal cord syndrome. Extradural lesions usually cause a wider distribution of pain, covering three to six dermatomes, while the intradural tumor may only affect one to two dermatomes.

It is estimated that 5% of patients with metastatic cancer will develop spinal cord compression. Kawabata et al. studied 3880 autopsy patients with a diagnosis of metastatic cancer. Two percent had clinical exam evidence of spinal metastasis, but the autopsy rate of metastatic lesions to the spine was 21–48%. In a study by Schaberg and Gainor of 322 patients with metastatic cancer, the rate of spinal metastasis was 2.2–31%. Breast, lung and prostate tumors were the most frequent tumors to cause spinal cord compression. Prostatic tumors were the most common cause of epidural impingement. Hypernephroma was the most common malignancy to present with neurologic impairment as the first clinical sign of malignancy.

In the present patient, the MRI scan revealed a mild compression fracture of T8 with infiltration of a gadolinium-enhancing mass into the paraspinal region as well as the T7 vertebra above and the T9 vertebra below. There was marked spinal cord compression at the T8 level and mild cord edema superiorly. A CT-guided needle biopsy showed malignant cells consistent with small cell carcinoma. He was transferred to the oncology service where he underwent debridement of the sacral pressure ulcer and received chemotherapy and radiation therapy for his lung cancer. He was transferred to the rehabilitation floor 2 months later, and was able to return home. Unfortunately, approximately 6 months after discharge he died as a result of his cancer.

Clinical Pearls

1. Early signs of a spinal cord tumor may mimic a variety of disease processes, so a high index of suspicion is needed if routine work-up is negative or treatment is unsuccessful.

2. Pain is an early presenting symptom of a spinal cord tumor, followed by neurologic signs of sensory loss and progressive weakness.

3. Extradural metastatic lesions of the spinal cord are the most common, so an increased risk of cancer should raise your level of awareness.

4. Extradural tumors are more aggressive and give a wider pain distribution compared to intradural tumors.

REFERENCES

1. Kawabata M, Sugiyama M, Suzuke T, Kumaro K: The role of metal and bone cement fixation in the management of malignant lesions of the vertebral column. Int Orthop 4:177,1980.
2. Ropper AH, Martin JB: Diseases of the spinal cord. In Wilson JD, et al. (eds): Harrison's Principles of Internal Medicine, 12th ed. New York, McGraw-Hill, 1991, pp 2080–2081.
3. Schaberg J, Gainor BJ: A profile of metastatic carcinoma of the spine. Spine 10:19, 1985.
4. Woods GW II: Other disorders of the spine. In Canale ST (ed): Campbell's Operative Orthopaedics. New York, Mosby, 1998.

PATIENT 67

A 70-year-old woman with headaches and back pain after a motor vehicle accident

A 70-year old-woman comes to your office for evaluation of headaches and progressive middle and low back pain that have been present since a motor vehicle accident 2 months ago. Her vehicle was struck obliquely from the front passenger side; her seatbelt was on, but broke loose at the time of impact, and she lost consciousness for less than 5 minutes. The patient has no complaints of arm or leg pain, paresthesias, or weakness. Back pain prevents her from sitting longer than 5 minutes, and she has to avoid repeated bending. She has had poor response to trigger point injections and physical therapy. Past medical history is notable for peptic ulcer disease and surgical menopause at 45 years of age. Current medications include H2 blockers, acetaminophen, and codeine for pain.

Physical Examination: General: alert, well developed, well nourished. Musculoskeletal: ambulates without antalgia; heel and toe walking intact; diffuse paraspinal tenderness most localized to upper lumbar segments. Spine: mild scoliotic deformity; increased thoracic kyphosis; lumbar forward flexion grossly restricted due to pain aggravation. Neurologic: reflexes intact at 1+ and symmetric; no ankle clonus or Hoffman's sign; muscle strength is 4+/5 throughout, without focal deficit.

Laboratory Findings (in emergency room): CT scan of head: negative. Cervical x-ray series: mild degenerative changes. Thoracic x-rays: chronic-appearing T1, T10, and T11 vertebral fractures, scoliosis, and osteopenia. No lumbar films were taken.

Question: What is the probable cause of her thoracolumbar pain?

Answer: Post-traumatic osteoporotic compression fracture

Discussion: Over the last decade, osteoporosis has become a major clinical challenge for physicians and patients due to the morbidity and mortality associated with fractures. The incidence of osteoporosis in postmenopausal Caucasian women in the United States is 21–30%. Approximately 1.5 million osteoporotic fractures occur per year in the U.S. One in two women and one in eight men over the age of 50 will suffer an osteoporotic fracture at some point. The economic cost of osteoporosis related to all fractures is 35–45 billion dollars per year. The lifetime risk of hip fracture in women is greater than the risk of breast, endometrial, and ovarian cancer combined. In men, the lifetime risk of hip fracture is greater than the risk of prostate cancer.

Osteoporosis is characterized by low bone mass and architectural arrangement deterioration, with a consequent increase in bone fragility and susceptibility to fractures. Osteoporosis has been classified into two categories: primary and secondary. **Primary osteoporosis** is subdivided into Type I and II. *Type I* is also known as post-menopausal or high turnover, and is due to decreased levels of estrogen resulting in increased activity of the osteoclasts and subsequent increased bone resorption. The female to male ratio is 6:1. The fractures are often noted in the vertebral body and distal forearm. *Type II* osteoporosis is also called senile type, or low turnover. There is cortical and trabecular bone loss, and the female to male ratio is 2:1. The fractures often associated with this type occur in the vertebral body, hips, pelvis, and long bones. **Secondary osteoporosis** is associated with bone marrow disorders, endocrine disorders, gastrointestinal disorders, connective tissue disorders, and other miscellaneous causes.

Osteoporosis is a painless condition often diagnosed after a painful insufficiency (atraumatic) fracture. Vertebral fractures, the most common osteoporotic fractures, may be spontaneous and may occur during an everyday activity such as rising from bed or while sitting down. Early intervention is the ideal management of osteoporosis. The consequences of osteoporotic fracture are chronic pain, kyphosis, loss of height, and loss of self-esteem. The fracture usually presents as an episode of acute localized pain, with or without trauma, in the mid-thoracic or lumbar region. Common presenting symptoms include paravertebral muscle spasm, limited spinal motion predominantly in the flexion plane, and increased pain with activity, particularly recumbency. It may also present as an acute hip fracture resulting in or after a fall.

The diagnosis of osteoporosis is made by measurement of the patient's **bone mineral density** (BMD). The National Osteoporosis Foundation guidelines recommend that bone mineral testing be performed on all postmenopausal women under age 65 who have one or more additional risk factors for osteoporosis, and all women aged 65 and older, regardless of risk factors. The World Health Organization defines osteoporosis using the BMD measurements. A BMD 2.5 SD below the young adult mean is considered osteoporosis. A BMD more than 1.0 SD below the young adult mean, but less than 2.5 SD below the mean, is considered low bone mass (osteopenia). The number of standard deviations above or below the mean for the young adult healthy population is referred to as the T-score. Even though radiographs are useful in evaluating for fractures and deformities associated with osteoporosis, the sensitivity is very poor for quantifying BMD. There has to be at least 30% loss of bone mass before radiographic evidence of low bone mass can be detected.

The techniques used for measuring BMD can be divided into those that measure bone density at central or peripheral sites. The central sites include the lumbar spine and the hip. Equipment that measures central BMD includes dual energy x-ray absorptiometry (DEXA) and quantitative computed tomography. The peripheral measurement can be obtained using single energy x-ray absorptiometry, peripheral DEXA or QCT, radiographic absorptiometry, or ultrasonometry. DEXA is probably the most commonly used technique to measure BMD, because of its ease of use, low radiation exposure, and its ability to measure BMD at both the hip and spine. Ultrasound densitometry of bone is a relatively new entry in the field of BMD measurements. Despite some limitations, there is a considerable strong potential for this technique due to the fact that it does not involve radiation exposure and can be easily performed in a primary care physician's office for screening large numbers of patients.

Note that the monitoring of serum or urinary markers of bone turnover may be useful in conjunction with a BMD measurement in the evaluation of response to treatment. However, it should *not* be used to diagnose osteoporosis, evaluate its severity, or select a specific treatment.

Patients should be educated in **lifestyle modification**, early weight-bearing and strengthening **exercise**, improving **coordination** and flexibility, **postural training**, and safety and fall prevention measures. Exercise that includes back strengthening, cardiovascular workout, and weight-bearing such as walking, jogging, and stair climbing have been shown to maintain as well as increase the bone mineral mass in osteoporotic patients. Weight-bearing exercises early in life increase bone mineral density and skeletal mass, thereby decreasing the incidence of fractures due to osteoporosis in later years. Modalities including ice, hot pack, and transelectrical nerve stimulation can also be useful in these patients. Abdominal binders and thoracolumbar orthosis may be helpful. Bracing with hyperextension braces such as the cruciform anterior spinal hyperextension or Jewett brace is helpful in patients with vertebral compression fracture due to osteoporosis. These braces limit flexion of the lumbar spine; such flexion adds pressure onto the end plates of already compromised vertebral bodies. Recently, vertebroplasty and kyphoplasty have been used for relief of severe pain as well as for restoration of some of the vertebral height loss due to osteoporotic compression fractures.

The following medications can **reduce bone resorption**:

• **Calcium** is the major inorganic component of bone. Sufficient calcium intake is critical during the skeletal growth period and decreases risk of fractures, especially of the hip. Dosage: 1200 mg/day for premenopausal women and 1500 mg/day for postmenopausal women. Side effects: constipation, digitalis toxicity, nephrolithiasis, and possible decreased bone turnover.

• **Estrogen** suppresses secretion of interleukin-6, increasing calcitonin synthesis. Side effects: increased risk of breast cancer or endometrial cancer with long-term usage. Close monitoring is required for patients with symptomatic gallbladder disease or chronic liver disease. Dosage: 0.625 mg/day in a cyclic fashion balanced by progesterone if intact uterus. If status post hysterectomy, than progesterone may not be needed.

• **Calcitonin** has an analgesic effect by stimulating endogenous opioids. It is available in both nasal and oral form and may be beneficial in patients who are not ideal candidates for estrogen therapy. Side effect: possible development of autoantibodies. Dosage: 50-200 IU/day for osteoporosis, 200 IU qod or three times a week for analgesic effect.

• **Bisphosphonate** binds to hydroxyapatite in bone. Once bound to mineralized bone surfaces, bisphosphonate inhibits osteoclastic activity 1000 times more selectively than osteoblastic activity. The net effect is new bone formation. Preparations include alendronate (5–10 mg/day) and risedronate (5 mg/day). Side effect: may cause esophageal erosions.

• **Vitamin D** can be obtained in the diet (fish oils, liver, and milk) or from sunlight-induced skin production. Dosage: 400-800 IU/day.

Medications prescribed to **increase bone formation** include:

• **Sodium fluoride** is the most potent stimulator of osteoblastic cells and increases trabecular bone density. It is not formally approved in the U.S. Side effects: nausea; gastric irritation including peptic ulcers; anemia; and arthralgias. Dosage: 25 mg/day with food, titrating up slowly over a few weeks.

• **Anabolic steroid** increases bone formation *and* decreases bone loss. Side effects: can lead to liver problems and masculinization. FDA does not approve it for osteoporosis.

In the present patient, the initial level of demonstrated pain and limitation suggested acute compression fracture, despite the initial plain film interpretation suggesting a chronic appearance. A subsequent radionucleotide bone scan demonstrated intense uptake at the T11 level consistent with that clinical suspicion. A sagittal T1-weighted thoracic MRI (see figure) revealed anterior wedging compression deformity at T11, with marrow edema suggesting an acute process. There was no evidence of bony retropulsion or spinal cord compression. A subsequent DEXA scan showed a T-score (bone mineral density in g/cm2 compared to young adult bone expressed in standard deviation above or below normal) of –3.98, which, in the presence of a compression fracture, is diagnostic for severe osteoporosis. The patient was treated conservatively with analgesics, physical therapy, and anti-reabsorptive agents to prevent/reverse bone loss and minimize the likelihood of further spinal fractures.

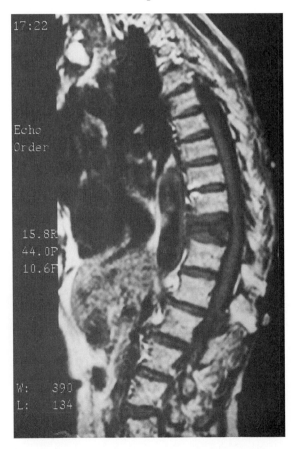

Clinical Pearls

1. The age of a compression fracture cannot be determined on plain films. Bone scan imaging and MRI provide added information in determining the acuteness of a vertebral fracture and therefore the probability of it as a source of acute pain.

2. The most common sites of vertebral fracture are low thoracic followed by high lumbar.

3. Consider treatment of osteopenia in the patient with risk factors as soon as loss of BMD below 1.5 SD is noted.

4. Weight-bearing exercise should be part of the comprehensive approach to treatment.

5. Osteoporosis is one of the leading causes of morbidity and mortality in the aging population.

REFERENCES

1. Cole HM (ed): Measurement of bone density with dual energy x-ray absorptiometry. JAMA 267:286–294, 1992.
2. Gamble CL: Osteoporosis: Drug and nondrug therapies for the patient at risk. Geriatrics 50:24–33 and 39–43, 1995.
3. Gosfield E III, Bonner FJ Jr: Evaluating bone marrow density in osteoporosis. Am J Phys Med Rehabil 79: 283–291, 2000.
4. Lane J, Riley EH, Wirganowicz PZ: Osteoporosis: Diagnosis and treatment. J Bone Joint Disease 78:618–632, 1996.

PATIENT 68

A 71-year-old man with a right above-knee amputation

A 71-year-old man underwent an above-knee (transfemoral) amputation 1 week previously as a result of diabetes complications. He was diagnosed with type II diabetes 10 years ago. Over the last 3 years, he became resistant to oral medications and has been using insulin. The patient's past medical history is also significant for coronary artery disease, peripheral vascular disease (for which a right femoral-popliteal bypass graft was performed 3 years ago), and a myocardial infarction that occurred 7 years previously. Prior to the amputation, the patient's functional abilities included household and limited community ambulation. He reports that he independently conducted his activities of daily living (ADLs) at home. He has a 20-pack year history of smoking, but quit 5 years ago. The patient is widowed and lives approximately 70 miles from the acute hospital.

Physical Examination: General: obese; no acute distress; stump wrapped figure 8 style, sutures present, no drainage. Cardiac: distant heart sounds. Chest: increased upper airway noise, but no crackles in bases. Skin: no ulceration in residual leg. Musculoskeletal: full passive range of motion with hip extension and flexion. Neurologic: 4/5 strength on right lower extremity hip adduction, abduction, and flexion; left lower extremity 4/5 throughout; standing balance fair (negative Romberg); decreased proprioception, two-point discrimination, and light touch in left foot; decreased memory. Patient transfers from supine to sitting with overhead trapeze.

Laboratory Findings: Hemoglobin 14 g/dl, BUN 22 mg/dl, creatinine 1.7 mg/dl, Hct 42%.

Question: Which prosthetic knee unit offers the best stability while standing?

Answer: Manual locking knee.

Discussion: The rehabilitation process of a patient with any amputation, but especially a transfemoral amputation, requires a comprehensive knowledge of the patient's preoperative functional status, his functional goals, and his energy requirements for ambulation. An amputee's prosthetic prescription depends on comorbidities and vocational/avocational interests.

The rehabilitation of amputees begins preoperatively with proper education on surgical techniques, prosthetic manufacture, and stump care. In this phase of rehabilitation, pre-prosthetic exercise programs to strengthen the intact leg, stretching to prevent flexion contractures, and training with appropriate assistive devices can begin.

Postoperatively, prosthetic fitting can be done within 2–3 weeks. Early fitting helps in facilitating early return to ambulation. Once the temporary prosthesis is completed, therapy can include pre-gait activities of balance and weight shifting on parallel bars. Although now most patients undergo outpatient therapy, it may be appropriate for elderly patients or patients with comorbidities such as cardiac disease to go into acute inpatient rehabilitation settings. Here, these patients can begin activities to ensure adequate functional levels for transfers, ADLs, and use of assistive devices for ambulation. Prosthetic training is advanced as tolerated, and the patient's potential for prosthetic use is evaluated by a physician well trained in the management of amputees.

Community reintegration including a formal driving evaluation should be done for those patients who display this potential. Hand controls or alterations in the gas and brake pedals are adaptations that can be evaluated in the rehabilitation setting. Special emphasis should be placed on vocational and avocational retraining as these activities seem to promote wellness, sociability, and improved aerobic fitness, which can improve overall functional ability. One study showed that patients who underwent inpatient rehabilitation retained their learned skills on 1-year follow-up. The initial investment of inpatient rehabilitation may show an advantage in overall functional outcomes.

An important component of the prosthesis in above-knee amputation is the prosthetic knee. Several types of prosthetic knees with specialized characteristics are worthy of discussion. The **manual-locking knee** usually includes a pull cord to unlock the knee for flexion in sitting. However, it does not allow for swing-phase knee flexion and is usually reserved for the elderly or debilitated patient for use only in transfers. The **constant-friction single-action knee** allows for free flexion and extension and is controlled by a friction unit that is adjustable. Single axis knees are durable and inexpensive; however, the patient may have problems with excessive heel rise in early swing phase and increased terminal swing impact with increased gait speed. The **weight-activated stance-control knee** or "safety knee" provides stable stance for up to 20 degrees of flexion. These knees function as a single-axis constant-friction knee during swing, but lock during stance when an axial load is applied. This knee is good for patients with mild pelvic weakness and for amputees needing stability on uneven surface. **Polycentric knees** incorporate a four-bar or six-bar design to allow rotational and translational motion about an instantaneous center of rotation. This type of knee unit has become increasingly popular. These are now more commonly used with an endoskeletal shank design. **Hydraulic and pneumatic fluid-control knee units** have been designed to provide resistance to knee motion that is proportional to walking speed. The Mauch SNS swing and stance fluid-control knee unit is an example of one of the more sophisticated units. This knee not only controls the knee velocity in swing phase, but also yields resistance to knee flexion during the stance phase as well. A unique property of this prosthetic knee unit is that it allows an amputee to walk downstairs one at a time without turning sideways.

Any evaluation of an amputee for functional prosthetic use includes an assessment of comorbidities. Amputees often have complicating factors of peripheral vascular disease, diabetes, and coronary artery disease, which can limit their ability to adequately use the prosthesis for functional ambulation. For the unilateral transfemoral amputee, the energy cost of ambulation is increased 40–65% above normal; the energy cost for a transtibial amputee is estimated to be only 9–28%. Because above-knee amputees are often elderly, not all will become functional community ambulators. Consider this when prescribing expensive prosthetic components. Prosthetic clinics offering the services of a physiatrist, certified prosthetist, and physical therapist can be very beneficial in counseling a patient on their potential with prosthetic use. This team approach ensures the formation of the most appropriate prescription.

Clinical Pearls

1. Rehabilitation of the amputee involves a multidisciplinary approach, with education and early evaluation of ambulation potential.

2. Numerous prosthetic knee units are available. They should be tailored to the functional capacity of the amputee.

3. Energy requirements for ambulation in the transfemoral amputee are greatly increased, warranting medical evaluation of comorbidities for appropriate prosthetic prescription.

REFERENCES

1. Braddom RL: Physical Medicine & Rehabilitation. Philadelphia, W.B. Saunders, 1996.
2. Delisa JA: Rehabilitation Medicine Principles and Practices, 3rd ed. (See Chapter 54, Table 54–5.) Philadelphia, Lippincott-Raven, 1998.
3. Kowalske PG: Daily functioning of patients with an amputated lower extremity. Clin Orthopaed Rel Res 361: 91–97, 1999.
4. Shurr DG, Cook TM: Prosthetics and Orthotics. Stamford, CT, Appleton and Lange, 1990.

PATIENT 69

A 45-year-old woman with extensive burns

A 45-year-old woman who lives alone in a high-rise apartment complex fell asleep while smoking, and the cigarette ignited her bed. The fire department arrived within minutes and was able to contain the fire and rescue the woman. She was immediately treated by the paramedics, who diagnosed her as having extensive burns to her torso and extremities and probable inhalation injuries. She was given face mask oxygen, intravenous lactated ringers, and morphine for pain, with every precaution taken not to compromise her respiratory status.

Physical Examination (in the emergency department):   Temperature 100.4°, pulse 120, blood pressure 110/78 mmHg, respirations 24. Skin: second- and third-degree burns on 45% of body surface area; anterior thorax and abdomen, both dorsal aspects of upper arms, dorsum of right forearm, and both anterior thighs involved. Cardiac: increased rate, regular rhythm. Chest: scattered ronchi, expiratory wheezing. Abdomen: hypoactive bowel sounds. Neurovascular: palpable radial and dorsal pedal pulses. Neurologic: difficult secondary to sedation from morphine and hydroxyzine; muscle stretch reflexes 2+ in upper and lower extremities; toes down-going on Babinski reflex; pupils equal and reactive to light.

Course: The patient required airway protection due to inhalational injuries, and she was intubated. Intubation also maintained normal respiration during IV pain medicine and sedation. Her wounds were coated with Silvadene, which acts as a broad-spectrum antimicrobial and helps to bring the eschar to the surface. Sterile gauze was lightly wrapped around the coated wounds to minimize contamination and loss of body heat. Emergency fasciotomies were unnecessary because none of her burns fully circumscribed her limbs or trunk. Once the patient was medically stabilized, she was transferred to a local burn unit.

Question: When should the burn patient start rehabilitation?

Answer: Rehabilitation is involved in the patient's treatment from the moment he or she arrives at the burn center.

Discussion: There are about 1.25 million burn injuries in the U.S. annually, resulting in 51,000 hospitalizations and 5500 deaths. The poor are at the highest risk for burn injuries. Seventy-five percent of deaths from burns result from house fires, and young children and the elderly are most at risk.

The rehabilitation doctor plays a major role in the treatment of the burn patient. Survival rates have increased for burn victims, and it is vital that these patients achieve the highest level of function and the best quality of life possible. The **multidisciplinary team approach** is especially critical in the care of burn patients. The team typically consists of the general and/or plastic surgeon, critical care specialist, physiatrist, nurses, dietician, physical and occupational therapists, respiratory therapist, psychologist, social worker, speech therapist, and orthotist.

Short-term goals are to control pain, maintain joint mobility, preserve strength and coordination, promote wound healing, encourage return to activities of daily living, and educate the patient and family. *Long-term goals* include minimizing scar formation and flexion-contractures, continuing strength and endurance training, teaching compensatory and adjustment skills, and reintegrating the patient into society.

The present patient received care from all of the team members mentioned above. A few of her rehabilitation issues will be addressed here. Physical and occupational therapies were instituted the day after she arrived at the burn center. Physical therapy concentrated on gentle range of motion, bed mobility, and transfers. She progressed toward a resistance exercise program using therabands. Note that range of motion is best performed during wound dressing changes, so that the therapist can evaluate the wounds at the same time and make adjustments to the therapy if needed. Because the patient underwent autografting of skin to her upper torso, it was vital that she re-establish regular range of motion in her shoulders when cleared by the plastic surgeon (post-graft day 4).

The occupational therapist worked in conjunction with the orthotist to instruct on proper body positioning and splinting. (It is wise to avoid the temptation to supply the burn patient with assistive devices because they discourage the patient from maximizing his/her own function.) Speech therapy helped the patient restore phonation, which had been weakened by her inhalational injuries. She was transfered to the acute rehabilitation service 1 week after grafting, and multidisciplinary care was continued. Two weeks later, she was discharged to home with outpatient therapy in place. Although she declined psychological support while in the hospital, she did opt for outpatient counseling and eventually returned to her job as a bookstore manager.

Clinical Pearls

1. There are approximately 1.25 million burn injuries in this country annually, accounting for 51,000 hospitalizations a year.

2. With a higher survival rate for major burn victims, the importance of the rehabilitation team in maximizing patient function and quality of life has received greater recognition.

3. The ideal time for the physical therapist to perform range-of-motion exercises is during wound dressing changes, because wounds can be evaluated at the same time, and therapy modified as needed.

4. The occupational therapist (OT) works closely with the orthotist, but in many institutions fabricates custom splints and orthotics without any need for outside help.

5. While there may be a natural tendency for the OT to supply the patient with assistive devices, instead the patient should be encouraged to maximize his/her own function independently.

REFERENCES

1. Brigham P, McLaughlin E: Burn incidence and medical care use in the U.S.: Estimates, trends, and data sources. J Burn Care Rehabil 17:95–105, 1996.
2. Constable JD: The state of burn care past, present, and future. Burns 20:316–324, 1994.
3. Spires MC: Rehabilitation of patients with burns. In Braddom RL (ed): Physical Medicine and Rehabilitation. Philadelphia, WB Saunders Co., 1996, pp 1215–1236.

PATIENT 70

A 38-year-old man with chronic low back pain radiating to the left leg

A 38-year-old man is referred for electrodiagnostic assessment of a possible lumbar radiculopathy. He has a history of chronic low back pain since childhood. During the month prior to the evaluation, he noted that the pain began radiating down his left leg into his foot. He has been participating in physical therapy, with mild improvement in his symptoms. He recently was diagnosed with L5-S1 spondylolisthesis on routine lumbar spine radiographs.

Physical Examination: Musculoskeletal: strength normal. Neurologic: sensory functions normal; deep tendon reflexes normal, except for decrease at left ankle.

Laboratory Findings: Nerve conduction study (left sural sensory and tibial motor): normal distal latencies, nerve conduction velocities, and amplitudes. EMG study: see table (*top*). H-reflexes: see table (*bottom*).

Question: Does this patient have a lumbar radiculopathy?

EMG Study

Muscle	Insertional Activity	MUAP Morphology	MUAP Recruitment
L VMO	Normal	Normal	Normal
L anterior tibialis	Normal	Normal	Normal
L medial gastroc	1+ fibs	Normal	Normal
L biceps femoris-short head	Normal	Normal	Normal
L gluteus maximus	1+ fibs	Normal	Normal
L lumbar paraspinals	1+ fibs/PSW	—	—

MUAP = motor unit action potential, VMO = vastus medialis obliquus, PSW = positive sharp waves, fibs = fibrillations

Tibial H-Reflexes

	H-reflex latency (msec)	H-reflex amplitude (mV)
L tibial	35.3	0.3
R tibial	31.7	3.5

Answer: Yes, a left S1 radiculopathy

Discussion: In the electrophysiologic diagnosis of a radiculopathy, there should be abnormalities present in two muscles innervated by the same nerve root, but by different peripheral nerves. No abnormalities should be found in muscles innervated by nerve roots adjacent to the abnormal one. Muscle sampling needs to be performed in muscles that are innervated just proximal and distal to the suspected level of injury. Electromyography evaluates the functional and physiologic integrity of the nerve better than imaging studies.

The most frequent cause of radiculopathies in patients less than 50 years of age is **nerve root compression by herniated disc**. In patients older than 50 years, the cause is most frequently nerve root compression due to degenerative changes in the spinal canal. Electrophysiologic changes due to a radiculopathy depend on the amount of pressure on the nerve root. When the pressure is severe enough to cause axonal loss, there is EMG evidence of denervation in the appropriate myotome. If the condition is chronic, the examination may only reveal evidence of reinnervation in the motor unit action potentials (MUAPs). If there is no evidence of denervation on the EMG, the radiculopathy may be causing only a focal compression that may or may not be associated with a conduction block.

Paraspinal muscles may show signs of denervation within 5–7 days of the onset of a radiculopathy. Examination of the paraspinal muscles gives little assistance in localizing the nerve lesion except to locate the lesion proximal to the plexus and affecting the posterior primary rami. The paraspinal musculature that is an exception to this rule comprises multifidus muscles, which are the deepest muscles in this area and the only ones considered to have monosegmental innervation. Multifidi examination techniques have been studied, but they will not be discussed here (see reference 2). Denervation changes in paraspinal muscles may also be caused by motor neuron disease, local trauma, metastasis to the posterior primary rami and paraspinal muscles, generalized myopathies, and diabetes mellitus. Peripheral muscles may not show abnormalities on EMG needle exam for up to 3 weeks after the onset of a radiculopathy. Needle electromyography will not be abnormal in presence of demyelinating lesion or conduction block unless the conduction block causes changes in the recruitment or interference pattern of the MUAP.

As in this case, motor and sensory nerve conduction studies (NCS) are usually normal in the presence of a single-level radiculopathy. Even if sensory loss is found clinically, findings on sensory NCS are rarely affected with radiculopathies because the lesion is preganglionic to the dorsal root ganglion. Motor nerve conduction velocities and distal latencies are typically normal because the lesion is a more central process and does not affect the peripheral nerve. Amplitudes of the compound muscle action potential (CMAP) may be affected if the radiculopathy is severe enough to cause significant axonal loss. Even if the axonal loss is severe, a decrease in the amplitude of the CMAP may not be appreciated because the peripheral nerves are comprised of nerve fibers from more than one nerve root.

H-reflexes may be valuable in assessing patients such as this one. Whereas needle electromyography only assesses the motor nerve, H-reflexes also evaluate the functioning of the sensory nerve fibers. Another benefit of the H-reflex is that it becomes abnormal early in the course of nerve root compression—even if the compression is not severe enough to cause axonal loss. Disadvantages of H-reflexes are that they can only assess a few nerve roots (S1 and C6/C7); they may be absent in normal patients over the age of 60; and they may not return to being normal or present once they are abnormal or absent from a previous injury. Moreover, abnormalities of the H-reflex are not specific for radiculopathies, but can also be due to peripheral neuropathies, plexopathies, and spinal cord dysfunction.

When bilateral H-reflexes are present, selecting the most meaningful H-reflex parameter for considering abnormalities is controversial. Parameters include side-to-side latency differences, absolute latencies normalized for age and leg length, absolute amplitudes, side-to-side amplitude differences, and amplitude ratio of symptomatic side to the asymptomatic side. Side-to-side differences in latencies of up to 1.8 millisecond are considered normal. H-reflex amplitudes are often smaller on the affected side. Amplitude ratio (amplitude of symptomatic side/amplitude of asymptomatic side) of less than 0.4 with normal differences in latencies is considered abnormal.

If the latency differences are within normal limits, but a S1 radiculopathy still is suspected, the use of the **amplitude ratio** to detect abnormalities is recommended. The ratio may be a good parameter when the radiculopathy is causing a conduction block in the absence of extensive demyelination. Using the amplitude ratio rather than the absolute amplitudes as a parameter is recommended because the amplitudes decrease with normal aging, but there is no age-effect on the ratio itself. Nor is the amplitude ratio affected by facilitation by isometric contractions. In a comparison study of S1 radiculopathies in 24 cases (documented by imaging studies) and 24 asymptomatic controls, the H-reflex amplitude ratio (asymptomatic/symptomatic) had 100% sensitivity and 95.8% specificity, compared with latency differences which had 95.8% specificity and 63.6% sensitivity. The authors concluded that when the H-reflex was present bilaterally, the amplitude ratio was more indicative of a S1 radiculopathy than latency differences.

In the present patient, the diagnosis was made based on the evidence of denervation in two muscles innervated by the S1 nerve root and the paraspinal musculature. Additionally, he had a significant H-reflex amplitude ratio.

Clinical Pearls

1. Evidence of denervation (such as the presence of fibrillations) on EMG in the paraspinal musculature supports the diagnosis of a radiculopathy.

2. For a single-level radiculopathy, denervation and/or reinnervation changes on EMG should be restricted to a single root level with abnormalities confirmed in at least two limb muscles innervated by different peripheral branches of that same nerve root.

3. Sensory nerve action potentials should be spared with preganglionic lesions (like a radiculopathy), but compound muscle action potentials may be affected by both preganglionic and postganglionic lesions.

4. Tibial H-reflexes are valuable for the diagnosis of S1 radiculopathies. They are abnormal early in the course of a radiculopathy, even if the compression does not cause axonal loss.

5. Amplitude ratio of the H-reflexes may be more sensitive to S1 radiculopathy than side-to-side differences in latencies, especially if the radiculopathy is causing a conduction block rather than extensive demyelination or axonal loss.

REFERENCES

1. Fisher MA: AAEM Minimonograph # 13: H-reflexes and F-waves: Physiology and clinical indications. Muscle Nerve 15:1223–1233, 1992.
2. Haig AJ, Parks TJ: Paraspinal muscles: Anatomy and electrodiagnostic testing in the cervical and lumbar regions. North Am Clinic Phys Med Rehabil 5:447–463, 1994.
3. Han TR, Paik NJ, Lim MS: Effect of facilitation and averaging on side-to-side H-reflex amplitude ratio (ab). Muscle Nerve 21:1580, 1998.
4. Jankus WR, Robinson LR, Little JW: Normal limits of side-to-side H-reflex amplitude variability. Arch Phys Med Rehabil 75:3–7, 1994.
5. Nishida T, Kompoliti A, Janssen I, Levin KF: H-reflex in S-1 radiculopathy: Latency versus amplitude controversy revisited. Muscle Nerve 19:915–917, 1996.
6. Wilbourn AJ, Aminoff MJ: AAEM minimonograph # 32: The electrodiagnostic examination in patients with radiculopathies. Muscle Nerve 21:1612–1631, 1998.

PATIENT 71

A 62-year old woman with left hemiplegia after radiation for a brain tumor

A 62-year-old woman was diagnosed with a glioblastoma multiforme in the right parietal lobe after a 3-month history of progressive clumsiness of the left hand. She did not have any weakness or numbness of the left side. A craniotomy was performed to remove the tumor. She did well postoperatively, and eventually received radiation therapy. The patient continued to do well until about 18 months later, when rapidly progressive weakness and numbness of the left side developed.

Physical Examination: Vital signs: normal. General: alert, oriented times three, normal speech and swallowing. Neurologic: mild left central facial weakness; all other cranial nerves grossly normal; sensation diminished to pinprick and light touch on left side, intact on right. Musculoskeletal: left upper and lower extremities 0/5, except for 1/5 left hip and knee extensors; right upper and lower extremities 5/5; muscle stretch reflexes decreased on left.

Laboratory Findings: MRI of brain: see figure.

Question: What condition is responsible for the patient's hemiplegia?

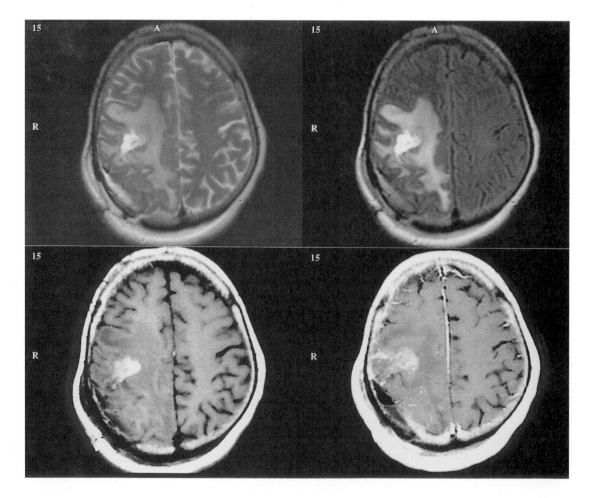

Diagnosis: Radiation-induced encephalopathy

Discussion: Patients who receive radiation therapy after surgery for a brain tumor can suffer from neurological injury from the radiation itself. Radiation-induced encephalopathy can be classified based on the time of onset of the symptoms (see table).

In the present patient, MRI confirmed focal cerebral radiation necrosis. She was given high-dose glucocorticosteroids, which instigated clinical improvement. The performance of stereotactic biopsy was essential, to allow differentiation of the radiation necrosis from tumor progression and to support a definitive diagnosis. This patient eventually underwent a craniotomy to remove the necrotic tissues.

The clinical and radiological presentations of early, delayed, radiation-induced encephalopathies may be difficult to differentiate from tumor progression or recurrence. MRI will show focal necrosis with or without edema, but this still may not allow differentiation. Positron emission tomography (PET) and single photon emission CT (SPECT) scanning can also be informative, since necrotic brain tissue has lower rates of metabolism compared to glial tumor tissues.

Syndromes Associated with Radiotherapy Toxicity

Radiation Syndrome	Onset after Radiation	Signs/Symptoms	Treatment	Comments
Early acute radiation reactions	Days	Headache Nausea/vomiting Fever Somnolence	Steroids	Responsive to steroids
Early delayed radiation reactions	Weeks to months (peak 1–3 mo)	Headache Somnolence	Steroids	
Late delayed radiation reactions				
Focal cerebral radiation necrosis	Months to years (peak 15–18 mo)	Focal neurologic findings of expanding mass lesion Worsening of pre-existing deficits	Steroids (high dose) Surgical debulking	Difficult to differentiate from tumor recurrence
Diffuse cerebral radiation injury	Months to years (peak > 12 mo)	Progressive dementia Psychomotor retardation Gait disturbance	Steroids	Incidence increases with radiation dosage and survival duration
Diffuse white matter leuko-encephalopathy	Usually > 1 yr	Lethargy, progressing to ataxia, dementia, death		Associated with concurrent methotrexate chemotherapy

From Bell KR, O'Dell MW, Barr K, Yablon SA: Rehabilitation of the patient with brain tumor. Arch Phys Med Rehabil 79 (suppl 1): S37–S46, 1998; with permission.

Clinical Pearls

1. PET and SPECT scans can help to differentiate tumor necrosis or progression from early delayed radiation reactions, because necrotic tissues have lower metabolic rates compared to glial tumor tissues.

2. Pathologic confirmation of a focal cerebral radiation necrosis is necessary for a definitive diagnosis.

REFERENCES

1. Bell KR, O'Dell MW, Barr K, Yablon SA: Rehabilitation of the patient with brain tumor. Arch Phys Med Rehabil 79 (suppl 1): S37–S46, 1998.
2. Kim EE, Chung SK, Haynie TP, et al: Differentiation of residual or recurrent tumors from post-treatment changes with F18-FDG PET. RadioGraphics 12:269–279, 1992.
3. Schwartz RB, Carvalho PA, Alexander E III, et al: Radiation necrosis vs. high-grade glioma: Differentiation by using dual-isotope SPECT with Tl and Tc-HMPAO. AJNR 12:1187–1192, 1991.

PATIENT 72

A 16-year-old girl with malnutrition, constipation, and amenorrhea

A 16-year-old girl with known cerebral palsy related to schizencephaly (neuronal migration defect) is admitted to the hospital for malnutrition, after a videofluoroscopic swallowing study demonstrated significant aspiration of all consistencies of food and liquid. She was treated for pneumonia a month prior. She has been followed for years in a specialty clinic, with frequent nutritional evaluations and provision of supplements. Her mother repeatedly denies any swallowing difficulty or pulmonary symptoms over these years, often saying, "She eats like a horse!" Her mother never consented to a swallowing study before the episode of overt pneumonia. The study was scheduled once, but the appointment was not kept because the family did not feel she had a problem in this area. Two years before this admission the patient required laparoscopy for bowel obstruction, and she is still troubled by constipation. She is amenorrheic and has been referred to adolescent medicine. Medications are Zantac, Robinul, Propulsid, iron sulfate, and Metamucil, all taken by mouth. Weight over the last year went from 19.6 kg to 22.5 kg, but progression from thinness to severe emaciation has resumed. The patient uses augmentative communication and has limited use of a gait trainer and stander, but is really dependent for all functional mobility and activities of daily living.

Physical Examination: Temperature 36.4°, pulse 112, respirations 20, blood pressure 101/76. General: weight 20.4 kg (representing a 4-lb weight loss since pneumonia 1 month ago); protrusion of known left dislocated hip as well as ribs and spine; almost no subcutaneous tissue (1 cm documented at most recent clinic visit); hydration clinically adequate. Musculoskeletal: mild kyphoscoliosis. Abdomen: overall soft and scaphoid; palpable stool, but no organomegaly. Chest: clear. Cardiac: normal.

Laboratory Findings: CBC: WBC slightly elevated; no lymphopenia. Chemistries: Na^+ 136 mEq/L, K^+ 3.3 mEq/L (low), Cl^- 87 mEq/L (low), CO_2 28 mmol/L, glucose 121 mg/dl, BUN 12 mg/dl, albumin 3.8 g/dl (borderline low), creatinine 0.6 µg/ml, zinc 0.69 µg/ml (borderline low) Chest x-ray: clear. Kidney/ureter/bladder x-ray: constipation. Shunt series: intact catheter. CT scan of head: no changes in ventricular size. Follow-through upper GI after videofluoroscopic swallowing study complete: see figure below.

Question: What major complicating gastrointestinal condition has developed?

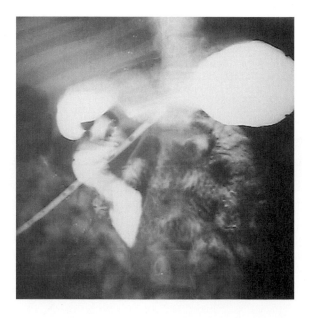

Diagnosis: Superior mesenteric artery syndrome

Discussion: This is superior mesenteric artery syndrome—not the atherosclerotic/vascular type, but the type with mechanical obstruction of the duodenum by the blood vessels when there is either extrinsic compression ("cast syndrome") or loss of the normal mesenteric fat pad in this area. The mechanism in this case is compression of the duodenum (see figure; note the sharp cut-off of contrast where the vessels cross the lower duodenum). The patient required and received urgent nutritional rehabilitation via **transpyloric tube feedings**, followed by placement of a **gastrostomy tube**. Her mother, who was fearful of surgery, struggled to avoid this for many years; she was willing to work very hard to nourish her child orally. The daughter had actually been referred twice for hip surgery and even been scheduled once, but the mother had cancelled the appointment.

The patient's mother also related that she had been told by a physician who helped originally diagnose her child with cerebral palsy: "Never let her get too fat—you won't be able to lift her." In retrospect, mediocre to inadequate weight gain was accepted for years, albeit with concern and attention, partly out of tolerance for parental preferences and biased reporting. Accepting 25th percentile weight for height has been recommended by some sources, but height and sometimes even arm span are difficult to measure and therefore not always obtained.

Laboratory evaluation should be considered; in this case, pre-albumin would have been helpful as it is more sensitive and specific than albumin or total lymphocyte count. **Decompensation** finally occurred with an episode of pneumonia. On follow-up, her weight was up to 23.7 kg.

The lack of prior serious pulmonary complications is also not uncommon; symptoms may be minimized, attributed to "sinus" or "allergy," and a good immune system and healthy lungs can clear and tolerate some influx of foreign material for awhile.

Superior mesenteric artery syndrome is also seen in the rehabilitation setting when there is substantial weight loss post trauma. In severe cases, there is copious gastric secretion that must be suctioned continuously, and prolonged nausea that responds partially to antiemetics. The syndrome may resolve either promptly or gradually as weight is regained via transpyloric tube feedings and/or hyperalimentation.

Clinical Pearls

1. Don't underestimate the emotional attachment to oral feeding and the desire to protect a child with a disability from pain and suffering.

2. Patients and families are remarkably poor at quantitation of actual food intake.

3. Never underestimate the persistent power of poor advice given sincerely to people in a state of heightened vulnerability. Deliberate malnutrition is a very bad substitute for good lifting techniques and equipment.

REFERENCES

1. Cambie M, Acerbi L, Bonora G, et al: The mesenteric artery syndrome. [in Italian] Pediatr Med Chir 5(1–2):115–118, 1983.
2. Samson-Fang LJ, Stevenson RD: Identification of malnutrition in children with cerebral palsy: Poor performance of weight-for-height centiles. Dev Med Child Neurol 42(3):162–168, 2000.
3. Vaisman N, Stringer DA, Pencharz P: Functional duodenal obstruction (superior mesenteric artery or cast syndrome) in cerebral palsy. J Parenter Enteral Nutr 13(3):326–328, 1989.

PATIENT 73

A 48-year-old man with tetraplegia and shoulder pain on change of position

A 48-year-old man suffered acute tetraplegia when a soft shoulder on the road he was driving gave way, and his logging truck rolled over. He was not restrained, and his head struck the top of the truck's cab, resulting in a C2 bipedicular fracture and evidence of a degenerative disc at C5–6. He was treated conservatively with halo fixation and transferred to an acute rehabilitation hospital. When rehabilitation was started, the patient noticed an aching and burning sensation in his right shoulder and arm that began approximately 10 minutes after sitting up and slowly became worse. It was relieved somewhat if he pulled his right arm close to his body and flexed the elbow, wrist, and fingers. However, after sitting up for 30 minutes, he needed to lie down, and the pain would slowly ease and improve over the next 10–15 minutes. If he sat back up, the pain would start again after 10 minutes. This was severely hampering his rehabilitation progress.

Physical Examination: Temperature 98.7°, pulse 82, respiration 14, blood pressure 110/64 HEENT: halo pin sites not infected; patient unable to move head in any direction, secondary to halo pins. Chest: clear. Cardiac: normal. Abdomen: nontender, with normal active bowel sounds. Musculoskeletal: full ROM of all joints in upper extremity except right shoulder, secondary to pain (when shoulder abducted/extended with elbow and wrist extended, "electrical" pains shoot down right arm and hand). Neurologic: hyperreflexic muscle stretch reflexes of brachioradialis and tricep bilaterally, and in lower extremities bilaterally; sensation impaired below C6 dermatomes, bilaterally; 5/5 strength in bilateral upper extremities with elbow flexion and wrist extension, 4/5 elbow extension, 1/5 strength with finger flexion, 0/5 strength with abduction of little finger, 4/5 strength in bilateral lower extremities with hip flexion, knee extension, and left ankle dorsiflexion, right ankle dorsiflexion 2/5, bilateral ankle plantarflexion 3/5. Rectal: normal sensation to pinprick and light touch, with weak but present voluntary anal sphincter contraction. Skin: normal.

Laboratory Findings: Hct 42.8%; platelets 164,000/µl. BUN 23 mg/dl, creatinine 1.1 mg/dl, albumin 3.2 g/dl. Urinalysis: normal. Cervical spine x-ray: see figure.

Question: What is the diagnosis?

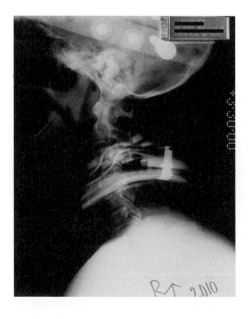

Diagnosis: Spinal cord stenosis at C5–6 vertebral disc with right C6 nerve root impingement when upright.

Discussion: Radiculopathy is pain in the distribution of a nerve root (in this case, the C6 nerve root). It may be associated with neck pain, sensory deficit, and motor deficiency. Pain production in a radiculopathy is multifactorial. Nerve roots may be directly compressed. Osteophytes, which develop as a reaction to the process of degenerative disc disease extending across the posterior and posterolateral aspect of the vertebral bodies, may cause compression or, as in this patient, may be secondary to a disc disruption. An inflammatory reaction may be a more significant cause of pain than actual mechanical changes. Studies have shown that compression of normal nerve roots results in paresthesias, while compression of an inflamed nerve root results in pain.

Perry and Nickels first used halo vest immobilization in 1959, after a cervical spine fusion in a patient with poliomyelitis. Complications have been reported: 36% pin loosening, 20% pin infections, 18% pin site pain; 11% pressure sore under the vest; disfiguring scar 9%; nerve injury 2%; dysphagia 2%. Halo fixation for 8–12 weeks may be sufficient to treat a cervical fracture with no compression of the neural elements. A rigid cervical halo for 8–12 weeks usually produces a stable, painless spine with minimal residual deformity and some loss of cervical range of motion. However, the elastic and plastic deformation that can occur to ligamentous structures and vertebral discs can lead to subacute instability; therefore, close monitoring is required. MRI has helped immensely in finding any ligamentous disruption after a spinal cord injury and is very helpful to the spine surgeon as he or she develops a treatment plan.

The present patient was initially treated with halo vest immobilization secondary to a C2 fracture with an incomplete injury. The C5–6 disc disruption was believed to be minor and not of great consequence, until rehabilitation was attempted. Pain was the main presentation and was associated with position—specifically, being upright. An MRI of the cervical spine was conducted because of the continued pain. The MRI showed a marked degeneration of the disc at C5–6, with a small to moderate right lateral disc herniation extending into the lateral recess and foramen. There was no sign of fracture at this level. There was also a focal area of increased signal density at the C5–6 level consistent with post-traumatic edema and myelomalacia.

Conservative management with oral steroids was elected, which allowed the patient to tolerate approximately 20 minutes of therapy before developing pain. When there was no significant improvement after 3 weeks, anterior cervical discectomy was performed at C5–6 with allograft bone. He was placed back in the halo vest for fixation and was able to return to rehabilitation unit 3 days later to resume his rehabilitation program. The pain in his right arm resolved, and he was able to participate well in therapy. The patient was discharged to home ambulating household distances.

Clinical Pearls

1. Nerve root compression can be minimal when supine, only to become clinically significant when in an upright position. In the present patient, the compression was probably secondary to the weight of the head and halo fixation device.

2. A trial of steroids can often mitigate the inflammatory response and decrease the patient's pain, allowing participation in rehabilitation.

3. If a conservative trial fails, then surgical correction with anterior cervical discectomy and fusion is often needed.

REFERENCES

1. Jones ET, Mayer P: The neck. In Weinsten SL, Buckwalter JA (eds): Turek's Othopaedics: Principles and Their Applications, 5th ed. Philadelphia, JB Lippincott, 1994.
2. Leventhal MR: Fractures, dislocations, and fracture dislocation of spine. In Canale ST (ed): Campbell's Operative Orthopaedics. New York, Mosby, 1998, pp 2714–2715.

PATIENT 74

**A 35-year-old man with severe low back pain and right leg radiation
after a motor vehicle accident**

A 35-year-old man presents with severe and disabling pain on the right side of his low back, with diffuse radiation to his right lower extremity. He has had no numbness or tingling in the extremities, and he has no complaints of weakness. His symptoms presented after a motor vehicle accident 12 weeks ago. At the time of the collision, his right leg was extended as he pressed the brake pedal.

Physical Examination: Vital signs: normal. Neurologic: 5/5 strength throughout upper and lower extremities; sensory intact to light touch, pinprick, and proprioception; tenderness localized in region of right posterior iliac spine; slight tenderness in right lower lumbar paraspinal musculature; reflexes symmetric bilaterally; long tract signs negative. Musculoskeletal: no pain in groin or back on Patrick's test; no pain in back or leg on straight leg raising test.

Laboratory Findings: X-rays of lumbar spine and pelvis: normal. MRI of lumbar spine, pelvis, and hips: normal,.CBC and SMA-7: normal.

Questions: Which procedure assists in obtaining the correct diagnosis? What is the diagnosis?

Answer: Fluoroscopically guided sacroiliac joint injection can confirm the diagnosis, which in this case is sacroiliac joint dysfunction.

Discussion: Sacroiliac joint pain remains a controversial source of extra-spinal low back pain. Sacroiliac joint pain is present in 13–30% of chronic low back pain patients. Many pain-sensitive structures exist in the hip and lumbar spine. Therefore, fluoroscopically guided injection is necessary to confirm that the sacroiliac joint is the primary source of pain.

Sacroiliac pain can be referred to the posterior iliac spine, lower lumbar region, buttocks, groin, medial and posterior thigh, lower abdomen, calf, and foot. It can be aggravated by sitting, riding, or bending, and is often relieved by standing or walking. It is often unilateral, but presents bilaterally in approximately 20% of patients.

The adult sacroiliac joint is C-shaped or auricular, with convexity facing anteriorly and slightly inferiorly. It is a diarthrodial joint because it contains synovial fluid; the articulating bones have ligamentous connections; the outer fibrous joint capsule has an inner synovial lining; and cartilaginous surfaces face each other, allowing motion. The ligamentous attachments include anterior iliolumbar and sacral ligaments, superior iliolumbar ligament, inferior iliolumbar ligament, and posterior sacroiliac, sacrospinous, and iliolumbar ligaments. The anterior blood supply is via the median sacral artery and lateral branches from the internal iliac artery; the posterior blood supply is by the gluteal arteries. The sacroiliac joint has diffuse anterior and posterior innervation. Posterior ligaments are supplied by the lateral branches of the posterior primary rami from L4-S3. The anterior innervation is from L2-S1.

Tenderness over the sacral sulcus and the posterior sacroiliac joint is common. Neurologic signs like motor weakness, sensory deficit, or neural tension are often absent unless there is a coexisting radicular pathology. Physical examination of the sacroiliac joint can be evaluated by several maneuvers, including the Gaenslen's, Patrick's, Yeoman's, Gillet's, sacroiliac joint shear, and standing and sitting flexion tests. Prospective studies show that these maneuvers do not confirm a diagnosis, but can (at best) enter the sacroiliac joint as a possible diagnosis.

The sacroiliac joint can be affected by certain rheumatologic diseases, such as ankylosing spondylosis, psoriatic arthritis, and Reiter's syndrome. Malabsorption disorders such as ulcerative colitis and Crohn's disease can also present with pain similar to that seen in sacroiliac joint dysfunction. Sacroiliac joint syndrome cannot be diagnosed by radiographic studies. Sacroiliac join injection under fluoroscopic guidance (see figure) remains the gold standard in diagnosis.

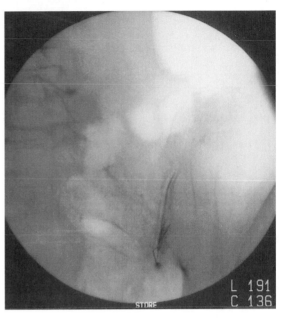

Fluoroscopic, contrast-enhanced sacroiliac joint injection.

The treatment goal is to restore the joint mechanics and overlying muscle function. Muscle imbalance can be addressed with joint mobilization, joint manipulation, and exercises. Sacroiliac joint injections under fluoroscopic guidance can be both diagnostic and therapeutic—and they have been used extensively in both regards. Radiofrequency ablation can help by denervating the posterior rim that supplies the joint. However, be aware that the sacroiliac joint does have innervation on the anterior aspect that cannot be approached with radiofrequency. Prospective studies are currently lacking in evaluating the efficacy of this procedure. A few case studies suggest that surgical fusion can sometimes be performed, but randomized controlled studies have not been done.

Clinical Pearls

1. The sacroiliac joint is a common cause of low back pain and can refer pain into the lower extremity.

2. The sacroiliac joint is a true diarthroidal joint that is innervated anteriorly and posteriorly.

3. Diagnosis is suggested by careful clinical history, physical examination, and ruling out other causes of low back pain, and is confirmed by fluoroscopically guided sacroiliac joint injection.

4. There are no pathognomonic laboratory or radiographic studies to diagnose the condition.

5. Presention can mimic symptoms seen in disc pathology.

REFERENCES

1. Bernard TN Jr, Casey JD: The Sacroiliac Joint Syndrome: Pathophysiology, Diagnosis, and Management. In Frymoyer JW (ed): The Adult Spine, 2nd ed. Philadelphia, Lippincott-Raven, 1997 pp 2343–2366.
2. Bogduk N: Clinical Anatomy of Lumbar Spine and Sacrum, 3rd ed. New York, Churchill and Livingston, 1997 pp 177–185.
3. Dreyfuss P, Michaelsen M, Pauza K, et al: The Value of Medical History of Physical Examination in Diagnosing Sacroiliac Joint Pain. Spine 21:2594–2602, 1996.
4. Fortin JD, Falco FJE: The Fortin Finger Test: An Indicator of Sacroiliac Pain. Am J Ortho 7:477–480, 1997.
5. Fortin JD, Kissling RO, O'Connor BO, Vilensky JA: Sacroiliac Joint Innnervation and Pain. Am Journal Ortho 12:687–690, 1999.
6. Mooney V: Understanding, Examining, and Curing Sacroiliac Pain. J Musculoskel Med 10(7): 37–49, 1993.
7. Moore MR: Outcomes of surgical treatment of chronic painful sacroiliac joint dysfunction. In Vleeming A (ed): Proceedings of the Third Interdisciplinary World Congress on Low Back and Pelvic Pain: The Most Effective Role for Exercise Therapy, Manual Techniques, Surgery, and Injection Techniques. Vienna, November 19–21, 1998. San Diego, University of California, Office of Continuing Medical Education, 1998, pp 218–226.
8. Schwarzer AC, Aprill CN, Bogduk N: The Sacroiliac Joint in Chronic Low Back Pain. Spine 20: 31–37, 1995.
9. Slipman CW, Jackson HB, Lipetz JS, et al: Sacroiliac Joint Pain Referral Zones. Arch Phys Med Rehabil 81:334–337, 2000.
10. Slipman CW, Sterenfeld EB, Chou LH, et al: The Predictive Value of Provocative Sacroiliac Joint Stress Maneuvers in the Diagnosis of Sacroiliac Joint Syndrome. Arch Phys Med Rehabil 79:288–292, 1998.

PATIENT 75

A 68-year-old man with swelling in his feet and ankles

A 68-year-old man notices swelling in both of his feet and ankles. He has not experienced recent trauma and does not have shortness of breath at any time of the day. He denies chest pain, fever, and chills. The edema reduces somewhat after he elevates his legs. There were no recent medication changes. His medical history includes non-insulin-dependent diabetes, osteoarthritis, and hypertension.

Physical Examination: Temperature 98.7°, pulse 74, respirations 18, blood pressure 154/95 mmHg. Oral cavity: no sputum or erythema. Cardiac: regular rate and rhythm; no murmur, gallop, or rub. Chest: no ronchi, wheezes, or rales. Abdomen: benign, no ascites or organomegaly. Neurologic: no focal deficits, but decreased sensation in a stocking distribution. Extremities: 2+ pedal and pretibial pitting edema; negative Homans' sign; nontender distal lower extremities; mild bilateral medial knee tenderness; crepitus with passive range of motion.

Laboratory Findings: Hct 31%, WBC 6800/µl, platelets 285,000/µl, Na^+ 149 mmol/L (normal 135–145), K^+ 5.5 mmol/L (3.3–4.9), uric acid 5.1 mg/dl (3–8 mg/dl). Urinalysis: trace glucose, rare WBCs, 2+ RBCs, no bacteria. X-rays: no acute or chronic abnormalities in ankles, but soft tissue swelling; moderate loss of medial joint space in knees bilaterally.

Question: What is the diagnosis?

Diagnosis: Acute renal toxicity (interstitial nephritis) secondary to chronic use of nonsteroidal anti-inflammatory drugs

Discussion: Much emphasis is placed on the gastrointestinal side effects of nonsteroidal anti-inflammatory drugs (NSAIDs), and the renal manifestations are often overlooked. The mechanism of injury to both the stomach and the kidneys involves one common factor: **inhibition of prostaglandin (PG) activity**. While certain PGs act as inflammatory mediators and play a role in the pain and swelling associated with osteoarthritis, PGs in the kidneys help with renal perfusion, and PGs in the stomach help maintain the protective barrier of the gastric mucosa.

The types of kidney damage that can result from NSAID usage include renal papillary necrosis, nephrotic syndrome, and acute interstitial nephritis. People who are at highest risk of kidney damage while taking NSAIDs include diabetics; those with underlying renal or hepatic disease, pyelonephritis, sepsis, or congestive heart failure; and those taking nephrotoxic drugs such as cyclosporins or aminoglycosides. Note that the present patient has both diabetes and hypertension.

A more comprehensive work-up in this case revealed serum BUN 55 mg/dl and creatinine 3.2 mg/dl (creatinine clearance was 23 ml/min—markedly reduced). Calcium and magnesium were normal. The patient was managed conservatively by discontinuation of the NSAID, careful hydration, sodium chloride restriction, and careful fluid input/output monitoring with the help of a Foley catheter. A diuretic was employed to help mobilize the edema in his legs and reduce his blood pressure; renal perfusion was maintained with the help of the IV fluids. He was started on clonidine (an antihypertensive medicine that does *not* reduce renal perfusion) 0.1 mg bid for hypertension control.

The osteoarthritis of the patient's bilateral knee medial compartment worsened as he became more active at home. His doctor prescribed celecoxib, which is selective for cyclo-oxygenase 2 (COX-2) inhibition. COX-2 is an enzyme that produces the PG which is found largely in inflamed joints and periarticular tissues; celecoxib does *not* inhibit COX-1, which produces the PG that helps perfuse the kidneys and protects the stomach. While COX-2 selective NSAIDs can still impair renal function and cause gastric and duodenal irritation, these effects are markedly less than the effects of nonselective NSAIDs.

A more recent trend is to use acetaminophen as a first-line drug for osteoarthritis of the knee. Many prospective, controlled trials have revealed that it is as effective as, and safer than, the traditional NSAIDs.

Clinical Pearls

1. Have a high index of suspicion for renal toxicity from NSAIDs when a patient develops hypertension, edema, and/or reduced urine output.

2. The mechanism of NSAID damage to both the kidneys and the GI tract involves inhibition of prostaglandin activity.

3. Kidney damage may be in the form of renal papillary necrosis, nephrotic syndrome, or acute interstitial nephritis.

4. Those at increased risk for NSAID-induced renal toxicity include patients with diabetes, hypertension, sepsis, congestive heart failure, pyelonephritis, or underlying renal or hepatic disease, and patients taking nephrotoxic drugs.

5. A recent trend has been to use acetaminophen as the first-line drug for osteoarthritis of the knee, because its efficacy equals that of ibuprofen and it offers better tolerance.

6. COX-2 selective NSAIDs are a safer alternative to nonselective NSAIDs because the former minimize harmful effects to the GI tract and kidneys.

REFERENCES

1. Bradley JD, Brandt KD, Katz BP, et al: Comparison of an anti-inflammatory dose of ibuprofen, an analgesic dose of ibuprofen, and acetaminophen in the treatment of patients with OA of the knee. New Engl J Med 325:87–91, 1991.
2. Brander VA, Oh TH, Alpiner N: Arthritis and connective tissue diseases. In Grabois M, Garrison SJ, Hart KA, Lihmkuhl LD (eds): Physical Medicine and Rehabilitation: The Complete Approach. Malden, MA, Blackwell Science, 2000, pp 1505–1533.
3. Miller SB: Renal diseases. In Woodley M, Welan A (eds): The Washington Manual, 27th ed. Boston, MA, Little, Brown and Company, 1992, pp 216–232.

PATIENT 76

An 80-year-old man with a numb hand

An 80-year-old man complains of numbness of his left hand (including the little finger), which has persisted for the past 6–7 months. He began noticing weakness of the left hand about 3 months ago. He denies any history of recent or remote trauma to either upper limbs. His past medical history is significant for coronary artery disease, hypertension, obesity, benign prostatic hyperplasia, and gastroesophageal reflux disease.

Physical Examination: Extremities: no remarkable joint deformity or swelling; Tinel's sign not elicited at elbow or wrist. Musculature: atrophy of first, fourth, and fifth dorsal interossei muscles; positive Froment's sign on left ; weakness of left abductor digiti minimi and left first dorsal interosseous; normal strength of remaining muscles, including flexor carpi ulnaris and flexor digitorum. Neurologic: sensation to both light touch and pinprick decreased on volar aspect of fifth finger.

Laboratory Findings: Blood and urine tests (screening for diseases associated with polyneuropathy): normal. Nerve conduction and EMG studies: see results below.

Question: What is the diagnosis?

Nerve Conduction Study

Nerves	Site	Distal Latency	Amplitude	CV
Sensory				
Left ulnar	Wrist	6.2 msec	0.3 μV	22.7 m/s
Right ulnar	Wrist	2.9 msec	7.3 μV	48.8 m/s
Motor				
Left ulnar	Wrist	4.4 msec	0.6 mV	—
	Below elbow	—	0.7 mV	55.4 m/s
	Above elbow	—	0.7 mV	20.4 m/s
Right ulnar	Wrist	2.5 msec	8.2 mV	—
	Below elbow	—	6.2 mV	50.1 m/s
	Above elbow	—	6.1 mV	51.4 m/s
Left median	Wrist	3.1 msec	5.2 mV	—
	Elbow	—	4.7 mV	45.5 m/s

CV = conduction velocity, m/s = meters per second
Ulnar nerve recording site: abductor digiti minimi
Median nerve recording site: abductor pollicis brevis

Left Ulnar Inching Test

Stimulation Site	Latency*	Latency diff.	Amplitude
Point 1	8.1 msec		0.66 mV
Point 2	8.6 msec	0.5 msec	0.50 mV
Point 3	11.5 msec	2.9 msec	0.71 mV
Point 4 1	2.1 msec	0.6 msec	0.88 mV
Point 5	12.7 msec	0.6 msec	0.88 mV

Point 1 = 4 cm distal to medial epicondyle
Point 2 = 2 cm distal to medial epicondyle
Point 3 = medial epicondyle
Point 4 = 2 cm proximal to medial epicondyle
Point 5 = 4 cm proximal to medial epicondyle
* Normal latency interval is < 0.6 ms

(Tables continued on next page.)

EMG Study

Muscle	Ins. Act	Fibs	PSW	Fascs	MUAP morph	IP
Left FDI	Reduced	1+	1+	None	Normal	Reduced
Left APB	Normal	None	None	None	Normal	Full
Left ADM	Reduced	1+	1+	None	Normal	Reduced
Left FCU	Normal	None	None	None	Normal	Full

Fibs = fibrillations, PSW = positive sharp waves, IP = interference pattern, MUAP = motor unit amplitude potential, FDI = first dorsal interosseous; APB = abductor pollicis brevis; ADM = abductor digiti minimi, FCU = flexor carpi ulnaris

Diagnosis: Left ulnar mononeuropathy at the elbow, with evidence of denervation

Discussion: Ulnar neuropathy at the elbow is the second most frequent entrapment neuropathy encountered in adults. Typical symptoms include numbness and tingling in the fourth and fifth digits; elbow pain or pain radiating from elbow into the ulnar aspect of the hand; and nocturnal awakening. Exacerbation of symptoms by elbow flexion or repeated wrist flexion may also be noted. Motor symptoms include an inability to adduct the fifth finger, weakened grip, and atrophy of the intrinsic hand muscles. In severe cases, an ulnar claw hand may develop. Neurologic examination may be normal in patients with intermittent symptoms that involve only the sensory component. Weakness of the first dorsal interosseous is more frequent than that of the abductor digiti minimi. In the absence of polyneuropathy, the muscle stretch reflexes are usually preserved. Tinel's sign over or proximal to the cubital tunnel may be elicited.

Several conditions predispose to ulnar nerve entrapment at the elbow, including congenital anatomical variations of the cubital tunnel, rheumatoid arthritis, uremic polyneuropathy, diabetic polyneuropathy, and elbow fracture or injury. There is an occupational predisposition to ulnar neuropathy at the elbow for professional musicians and athletes.

Electrodiagnostic examination is necessary to identify the site of lesion and rule out other causes mimicking the symptoms. The differential diagnosis of ulnar neuropathy includes C8 radiculopathy, lower trunk or medial cord plexopathy, polyneuropathy, carpal tunnel syndrome, and central nervous system lesions such as cerebral infarction or amyotrophic lateral sclerosis.

Electrodiagnostic exam should include an ulnar sensory and motor nerve conduction study (NCS). If this is abnormal, further NCSs should include the median nerve and the contralateral ulnar nerve for comparison, to exclude a diffuse process. The ulnar NCS should be performed with the patient's elbow in moderate elbow flexion (70-90° from horizontal). If ulnar motor NCSs recorded from the abductor digiti minimi are inconclusive, further testing may be done with recordings from the first dorsal interosseous muscle. An **ulnar inching study** (with stimulations 1–2 centimeters apart around the cubital tunnel) that assesses for changes in compound motor action potential amplitude or area, or abnormal latency differences, may help localize the lesion. Depending on the results of NCSs, needle electromyography may be indicated. EMG examination should always include the first dorsal interosseous muscle (the most frequent muscle to demonstrate abnormalities in ulnar neuropathy at the elbow) and ulnar-innervated forearm flexor muscles. If ulnar innervated muscles are abnormal, examination should be extended to include non-ulnar C8, medial cord, and lower trunk innervated muscles and cervical paraspinals to exclude brachial plexopathy and radiculopathy.

Other diagnostic tests, which may be useful, include plain radiographs of the elbow to identify old fracture, deformity, arthritic changes, and the rare congenital anomaly "ligament of Struthers" with associated bony spur.

Treatment of ulnar neuropathy at the elbow includes both conservative and surgical strategies. Nonoperative treatment includes educating the patient to avoid pressure on the elbow and prolonged elbow flexion; modifying the work environment; and splinting the elbow during sleep to discourage prolonged flexion. Patients who demonstrate fixed sensory loss and pain, weakness, or significant denervation on electrodiagnostic exam should be considered for surgical treatment. The most common surgical approach is decompression of the nerve at the elbow, but there is no consensus as to the optimal surgical method.

Patients exhibiting intermittent, sensory-only symptoms have a good prognosis with conservative management. The most consistent predictor of good outcome is the duration of symptoms before surgery. Most reports in the surgical literature are optimistic, with satisfactory improvement or complete recovery achieved in 80–90% of patients undergoing decompression by a variety of means.

In the present patient, clinical history and exam encouraged a suspicion of ulnar neuropathy. The site of injury was localized by electrodiagnostic exam to the elbow. The needle EMG also revealed significant axonal loss and denervation of ulnar innervated hand intrinsic muscles.

Clinical Pearls

1. Ulnar neuropathy at the elbow is common and may be the presenting manifestation of various medical conditions. The differential diagnosis includes C8 radiculopathy, lower trunk or medial cord plexopathy, carpal tunnel syndrome, polyneuropathy, and central nervous system lesions like cerebral infarction and amyotrophic lateral sclerosis.

2. Ulnar neuropathy may be predisposed in certain occupations (e.g., musicians and athletes) and in musculoskeletal changes at the elbow joint such as those due to trauma or fractures.

3. Clinical diagnosis is suggested by the history and physical exam. Localizing the lesion is facilitated by electrodiagnosis, but the diagnosis may be missed in mild cases with intermittent, sensory-only symptoms.

4. Treatment of ulnar neuropathy at the elbow can be conservative or surgical. Mild cases improve significantly with conservative management. Patients with denervation or fixed sensory or motor loss may benefit from surgical decompression.

REFERENCES

1. American Association of Electrodiagnostic Medicine, American Academy of Neurology, American Academy of Physical Medicine and Rehabilitation: Practice parameter for electrodiagnostic studies in ulnar neuropathy at the elbow: Summary statement. Muscle Nerve 22(3):408–11, 1999.
2. Bradshaw DY, Shefner JM: Ulnar neuropathy at the elbow. Neurol Clin 17:447–61, 1999.
3. Campbell WW: Ulnar neuropathy at the elbow. Muscle Nerve 23(4):450–452, 2000.

PATIENT 77

An 85-year-old woman with right hemiplegia and an inability to communicate

An 85-year-old woman with right-sided weakness and inability to talk was diagnosed with a large middle cerebral artery stroke on the left. She was initially lethargic, but showed gradual clinical improvement to the point that she was able to participate in rehabilitation about 1 week after the onset of her stroke.

Physical Examination: Blood pressure 155/70, pulse 90, respiration 18, temperature 97.7°. General: alert, no acute cardiorespiratory distress. Cardiac, chest, abdomen: normal. Extremities: no edema or redness. Neurologic: alert, able to follow one- to two-step commands, cooperative; speech fluent, nondysarthric, no hypophonia; unable to repeat words, but positive for word finding; naming deficits present. Cranial nerves: right lateral gaze palsy, right central facial weakness, tongue midline, hearing intact; sensation absent on right. Musculoskeletal: right hemiparesis, 0/5 upper extremity strength, 1/5 lower extremity strength; muscle stretch reflexes increased on right.

Question: What kind of language disorder does the patient have?

Answer: Conduction aphasia

Discussion: Aphasia is defined as the absence or impairment of the ability to communicate through speech, writing, or signs due to pathology in the language areas of the brain. It is important to determine the difference between fluency aphasia and psychotic speech. A patient with true aphasia also has other neurological deficits, such as hemianopsia, dysphagia, and hemiparesis.

The different types of aphasia are commonly classified based on a system associated with the Boston School of Aphasia (see figure). This classification uses fluency, comprehension, repetition, and word finding to determine the type of aphasia afflicting a patient.

The presence of fluency and apparent ability to comprehend, together with the inability to repeat words and to name objects, as seen in the present patient, is descriptive of **conduction aphasia**. This syndrome is due to a lesion in the arcuate fasciculus,

which is a structure connecting **Wernicke's and Broca's areas**. When an individual hears a word, Wernicke's area receives the output the word generates from the primary auditory area of the cortex. From there, the pattern is transmitted by the arcuate fasciculus to Broca's area. The articulated form of the word is then aroused in Broca's area, and passed on to the motor area of the cortex, which controls the muscles of speech. If the spoken word is to be spelled, the auditory pattern is passed on to the angular gyrus, where the visual pattern is elicited.

The present patient was treated with the stimulation-facilitation technique. A functional approach was used, combining speech, gesture, drawing, and mime. More recently, computer-based interactive technology has been applied to improve language function in chronic aphasia.

Diagnostic Schema for Classification of Aphasia

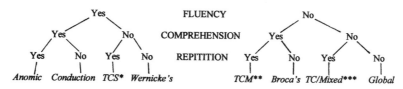

Legend:
*   *TCS* - Transcortical Sensory
**   *TCM* - Transcortial Motor
***   *TC/Mixed* – Transcortical/Mixed

Clinical Pearls

1. Test for fluency, comprehension, repetition, and word finding to determine the type of aphasia a patient has.

2. It is important to distinguish psychotic speech from fluent aphasia—a patient with the latter has associated neurological deficits.

REFERENCES
1. Aftonomos LB, Steele RD, Wertz RT: Promoting recovery in chronic aphasia with an interactive technology. Arch Phys Med Rehabil 78:841–846, 1997.
2. Kirsteins AE, Black-Schaffer RM, Harvey RL: Stroke Rehabilitation. 3. Rehabilitation Management. Arch Phys Med Rehabil 80:S-17, 1999.
3. Tippett DC: Speech-language pathology evaluation and treatment. In O'Young B, Young MA, Stiens SA (eds): PM&R Secrets. Philadelphia, Hanley & Belfus, 1997.

PATIENT 78

A 7-year-old girl with Cockayne syndrome, severe weight loss, and difficulty walking

A 7-year-old girl is followed for habilitation needs through an outreach clinic. She is known to have Cockayne syndrome, an autosomal recessive disorder, with typical features such as microcephaly, developmental delay, hearing impairment and language delay, poor weight gain, hand deformities, multiple joint contractures, and parchment-like skin. At a visit when she was 21 months of age, she was taking a bottle (which you advised discontinuing) and had gained a few pounds in the past 12 months. She took a few steps with help and reached out to grasp objects with either hand. She was alert and sociable. She was not toilet-trained, and you advised beginning this process. She had "mild increased tone" in the lower extremities. Her fontanel was delayed in closing, and she had mild frontal bossing. The geneticist considered her hand deformities, with MCP and DIP **hyperextension** ("swan neck"), unusual. She did not have cataracts.

At that time, the patient received hand surgery and splinting, as well as occupational, physical, and speech and language therapy at a local developmental center. The center's staff gave her a receptive age of 17 months and an expressive age of 12 months; her family indicated that she was doing better with the therapy, and they understand her more readily. She learned to feed herself in the subsequent year, and progressed to cruising and later independent ambulation with a walker or with one person holding her hand a few months before her third birthday. Her weight gain was limited but consistent. By age 3, she reportedly was telling her family when she needed a diaper change, but never did become truly continent.

Between ages 5 and 6, she was being seen about every 6 months; during this period she seemed to stop making progress and for the first time actually lost weight. She was described as "absolutely emaciated . . . other children in family well nourished to obese." Neglect was suspected as there were unused cases of Pediasure (liquid nutrition) in the home, per report. A pediatrician recommended she go back to bottle feeding.

The patient's therapy has been sporadic since transfer to public school. She takes a few steps in a very crouched position with help and rarely uses the walker. Weight varies up and down by a pound or two; more supplements and a power wheelchair are prescribed. She is more inconsistent about telling family about needs to urinate, and attempts at training are abandoned. A different physiatrist saw her at the time of wheelchair fitting and noted that her reflexes were "brisk throughout." At 7 years of age, when she does not walk at all in clinic though she is said to at home, the level of concern is very high, and a more detailed examination is conducted.

Physical Examination: General: weight 24 pounds (does not appear emaciated, but very thin); hydration clinically adequate; urinary odor suggests infection. Neuromuscular: lower extremity muscles atrophied; on supported standing, she hyperextends rather than flexes right knee; knee jerk very brisk; tight heel cord on right, with several beats of clonus and upgoing toe; left side not as abnormal, with few beats of clonus at ankle, +2 knee jerk, and equivocal Babinski reflex. She has never been verbal enough to give anyone a good sensory exam, and today is no exception. HEENT: jaw jerk not brisk; head on neck posture abnormal; dental caries present. Extremities: hands mostly unchanged, except for some increased stiffness of right-side deformities. Abdomen: benign without masses, other than some palpable hard stool. Chest: clear. Cardiac: no abnormal sound.

Laboratory Findings: Urinalysis with culture and sensitivity: urinary tract infection confirmed. CT scan of head, genetics follow-up, audiology testing, and urodynamics study: appointments missed because these must be done at a central location rather than locally, and the family can afford only a few trips. In addition, their only vehicle has now broken down.

Question: You talk with the social worker and nurses and they can arrange for transportation for one trip to the main pediatric hospital in the near future. What tests are most critical to schedule as top priority?

Answer: Brain and cervical spine MRI

Discussion: MRI of the brain and cervical spine (see figure) demonstrate markedly decreased volume of the splenium and corpus callosum (typical of Cockayne syndrome), but no hydrocephalus or other abnormality in the head; however, there is marked cervical canal narrowing with CSF effacement and impingement of the upper cervical cord. Although **hyperreflexia** is commonly noted in Cockayne syndrome, it usually goes along with other signs of cerebral dysfunction and is not known to be due to spinal cord pathology; nor is it reported to be so dramatically progressive, and

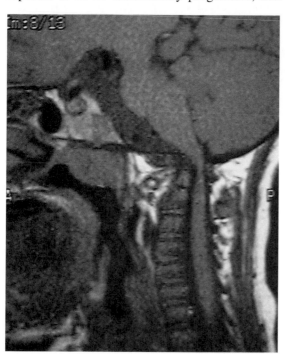

flexion contractures are expected rather than any **hyperextension**. The **asymmetry** was also a good clue to spinal cord injury (in the absence of a stroke syndrome or other unilateral trauma), as Cockayne syndrome is a symmetrical condition. Neurogenic bladder and bowel may be more difficult to evaluate in a developmentally incontinent child, but in this case significant indications were there when a detailed history was more carefully considered. In retrospect, **cervical dysphagia** may have caused her weight loss.

The author has also seen cervical dysphagia in a school-aged girl with mixed spastic/dystonic cerebral palsy, whose swallowing and nutritional status deteriorated without any change in her shunted hydrocephalus or periventricular leukomalacia, and whose cervical spine problem was diagnosed later after susbstantial pulmonary and urologic deterioriation and loss of other limited motor control that she had. Additionally, spinal cord injury is sometimes superimposed on the disability of young people with arthrogryposis, juvenile rheumatoid arthritis, Down syndrome, and other conditions that can affect the cervical spine.

The present patient receives spinal decompression and stabilization just 1 month before her seventh birthday. A year later, she weighs 26 pounds and is functional again, but is back to walking in a fairly crouched position. One contributing cause is hip flexion contractures resulting from inadequate therapy due to personnel shortages locally. The Babinski reflexes are unchanged, but the marked hyperreflexia is gone, and she has increased muscle bulk in both legs. The family really is not pushing her toilet training, but there are no further urinary tract infections.

Clinical Pearls

1. Even in the face of known progressive diseases, there may be aspects of a person's total condition that are highly treatable, and of which recognition and managment can offer great benefit. These aspects should not be accepted as part of the underlying disorder.

2. Blaming a family for poor progress, especially one that cares enough to keep bringing a child back to clinics, can be a huge mistake! Give the benefit of the doubt and look for other problems first.

REFERENCES

1. Kidron D, Steiner I, Melamed E: Late-onset progressive radiculomyelopathy in patients with cervical athetoid-dystonic cerebral palsy. Eur Neurol 27(3):164–166, 1987.
2. Mathews JA: Wasting of the small hand muscles in upper and mid-cervical cord lesions. QJM 91(10):691–700, 1998.
3. Nance MA, Berry SA: Cockayne syndrome: Review of 140 cases. Am. J. Medical Genetics 42:68–84, 1992.
4. Zeidman SM, Ducker TB: Rheumatoid arthritis: Neuroanatomy, compression, and grading of deficits. Spine19(20): 2259–2266, 1994.

PATIENT 79

A 19-year-old man with tetraplegia and headache with micturition

A 19-year-old man dove into shallow water, hit his head, and immediately experienced upper and lower extremity weakness. He underwent open reduction and internal fixation of a C5–6 fracture dislocation with anterior cervical discectomy and fusion from C4 to C7. He regained elbow flexor and wrist extensor strength consistent with a C6 complete spinal cord injury, and was transferred to an acute rehabilitation hospital. The patient progressed well, and on discharge to home he was reflex voiding using a condom catheter with low post void residuals. He now returns to see you in clinic. He reports he is doing well at home, but is experiencing headaches when he voids. He describes the headache as a pressure behind his eyeballs. He also reports mild facial and upper chest sweating with each episode.

Physical Examination: Temperature 99.2°, pulse 70, respiration 16, blood pressure 95/64. HEENT: cervical collar in place. Chest: clear. Cardiac: normal. Abdomen: mildly distended; nontender, with normal active bowel sounds. Musculoskeletal: full range of motion of bilateral upper extremities with no shoulder pain; tightness developing with mild contractures at hip, knees, and ankles. Neurologic: hyperreflexic muscle stretch reflexes with flexor spasms of bilateral lower extremities on minimal stimulation; 5/5 strength in bilateral elbow flexors; 4/5 strength in bilateral wrist extensors; 0/5 strength with bilateral elbow extension, finger flexion, and abduction of little finger; 0/5 strength in bilateral lower extremities. Skin: red but blanchable skin over sacral area. Rectal: positive bulbocavernosa reflex, no sensation to pinprick or light touch, no voluntary muscle contraction.

Laboratory Findings: CBC and chemistries: normal. Urinalysis: pH 7.0, specific gravity 1.020, blood negative, leukocyte esterase negative, nitrate negative, occasional WBC, occasional bacteria. Cystogram: see figure.

Question: What is the diagnosis?

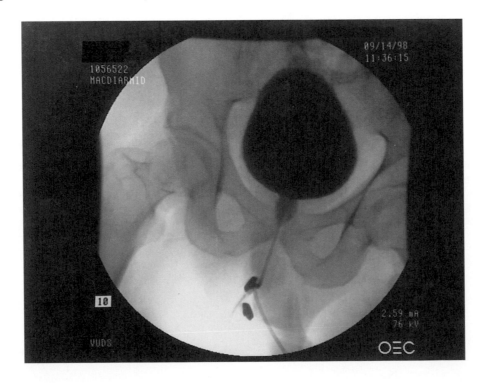

Diagnosis: Detrusor-external sphincter dyssynergia with autonomic dysreflexia.

Discussion: Detrusor-external sphincter dyssynergia (DESD) occurs commonly after a suprasacral spinal cord injury and refers to the failure of the external urethral sphincter to relax during bladder contraction. Because of the high intravesical pressure that results, 50% or more of patients afflicted with DESD suffer long-term urological complications. The problems associated with DESD are not only recurrent urinary tract infections, but vesicoureteral reflux, hydronephrosis, urinary calculus formation, and renal insufficiency or failure.

Autonomic dysreflexia (AD) is a syndrome that can be life threatening to an individual with a spinal cord injury, and is the result of massive paroxysmal reflex sympathetic activity. AD presents with paroxysmal hypertension with resultant pounding headaches, visual disturbances, and/or chest pain. It occurs most commonly in individuals with an injury at the T6 level, which is above the major splanchnic sympathetic outflow, but has been reported in patients as low as the T8 level. The most frequent trigger of AD is a noxious stimulus below the level of injury.

Bladder distention accounts for 75–85% of episodes of AD. The second most common trigger is **bowel distention** due to fecal impaction. After an initial period of spinal shock, AD can appear anytime from 2 months to 13 years after a SCI, but most commonly within 6 months. The present patient was experiencing bladder distention due to DESD and the resultant symptoms of headache and elevated blood pressure. The triad of headache, sweating, and cutaneous vasodilatation has been reported in 85% of studies.

Treatment of DESD varies based on the needs and preferences of the patient. Use of anticholinergics to relax the bladder plus intermittent catheterization to empty the bladder is one method. Dantrolene or baclofen to relax the skeletal muscle of the external sphincter or an alpha-blocker to relax the bladder neck is often helpful. An indwelling Foley catheter can also be used to drain the bladder and prevent high bladder pressures. Surgical management options are:

1. Sphincterotomy to reduce the outlet resistance and a condom catheter with a leg bag

2. Suprapubic catheter with a leg bag

3. Intraurethral stent prosthesis to keep the urethral sphincter open, with condom catheter and leg bag

4. Dorsal rhizotomy of the sacral roots and placement of a sacral root electrical stimulator

5. Bladder augmentation with continent or incontinent stoma.

Selection of a management option should occur only after discussing all the options with the patient, but it is best to start with the most conservative approach.

In the present patient, the cystogram revealed that the bladder was contracting and the bladder neck was open, but the external sphincter was not relaxing. This state caused filling of the prostatic urethra with intravesicular cutoff at the level of the external sphincter. After discussion of all the options, the patient chose oxybutynin with intermittent catheterization. His headaches resolved.

Clinical Pearls

1. Detrusor-external sphincter dyssynergia (DESD) is common in suprasacral spinal cord injury and can lead to a high-pressure bladder system and renal deterioration if not treated.

2. DESD can present with the clinical symptoms of autonomic dysreflexia (AD)— a triad of headache, sweating, and skin vasodilatation—when the patient spontaneously empties his or her bladder.

3. Treatment of DESD varies, but the key is to prevent high bladder pressures and minimize risk of urinary tract infections. Treatment decisions can be made only after discussing all of the options with the patient.

REFERENCES
1. Juan Garcia FJ, Salvador S, Montoto A, et al: Intraurethral stent prosthesis in spinal cord–injured patients with sphincter dyssynergia. Spinal Cord 37:54–57, 1999.
2. Lee BY, Karmakar MG, Herz BL, Sturgill RA: Autonomic dysreflexia revisited. J Spinal Cord Med 18:75–87, 1995.

PATIENT 80

A 67-year-old man with a right transtibial amputation and a swollen stump

A 67-year-old man had a right transtibial (below-knee) amputation 3 years ago because of peripheral vascular disease. He has been using a prosthesis with a silicone gel liner and has been independent in his ambulation, using a straight cane only on uneven surfaces. About 8 months ago, gradually increasing pain and swelling in his stump developed. Review of systems is significant for weight gain of about 15 pounds.

Physical Examination: Vital signs: normal. General: alert; oriented to person, place, and time; no acute distress; ambulated and transferred well independently with prosthesis. Extremities: right lower transtibial amputation; residual limb measuring five inches long, with healed linear myoplasty scar; hyperpigmentation, thickening, and +1 edema at distal end. Musculoskeletal: 4+/5 to 5/5 strength in all extremities, including residual limb.

Question: To what condition can these findings be attributed?

Answer: "Choked stump" syndrome

Discussion: Choked stump syndrome pertains to a condition caused by poor socket fit in a patient with a lower extremity amputation. When the socket is tight in a circumferential manner around the proximal part of the residual limb (e.g., when the patient gains weight), edema and tenderness result at the distal end, where there is lack of contact between the residual limb and the socket. There is usually a discernible area of constriction delineating the margin of edema.

If the proximal constriction is not alleviated, the edema leads to stretching and induration of the skin. Because of obstruction to venous outflow, erythema can also be seen. Later on, deposition of hemosiderin from extravasated red blood cells leads to hyperpigmentation of tissues, which is usually permanent. Eventually, the combination of stasis pigmentation, hemorrhagic papules, and nodules gives the tissues involved a verrucous appearance.

The present patient's weight gain was causative in this case. Treatment of the choked stump syndrome is relief of the proximal constriction and restoration of total contact between the residual limb and socket, especially at the distal end.

Clinical Pearls

1. Well-delineated swelling in a lower extremity amputation residual limb, long after complete wound healing has occurred, is indicative of choked stump syndrome.

2. A verrucous and hyperpigmented appearance of the skin of a residual limb (as in the present patient) are reliable signs that the edema and constriction are chronic.

REFERENCES

1. Eftekhari N: Amputation rehabilitation. In O'Young B, Young MA, Stiens SA (eds): PM&R Secrets. Philadelphia, Hanley & Belfus, 1997, pp 214–222.
2. Leonard JA, Meier RH: Upper and lower extremity prosthetics. In Delisa JA, Gans BM (eds): Rehabilitation Medicine: Principles and Practice, 3rd ed. Philadelphia, Lippincott-Raven, 1998, pp 669–696.

PATIENT 81

A 15-year-old girl with ataxia, weakness, and progressive mental status changes

A 15-year-old girl experienced 2 weeks of worsening headache and neck pain before admission to an acute care service due to seizure activity. She was bitten by a tick 3–4 weeks prior. She is now taking Ativan and Dilantin. Her past history is remarkable for abuse by a stepfather and some right-sided hearing problems, but she is a popular young woman and makes good grades in regular classes. Nine days after admission you are asked to consult on inpatient rehabilitation, because she continues to demonstrate confusion and other mental status changes.

Physical Examination: Afebrile, blood pressure 120/60, pulse 80, respirations 16. Neurologic: alert and oriented to person and season of year only; follows one-step commands with cues; repeats phrases such as "mommy, yes" and "I'm pretty, I'm not pretty" incessantly, but no other suggestion of delusion or hallucination; diffusely brisk reflexes, but no clonus and equivocal Babinski reflexes; difficulty with finger-to-nose testing; wide-based, unsteady gait, with head down. Cranial nerve and funduscopic exam: normal; extraocular muscles intact. Musculoskeletal: full range of motion throughout; no arthropathy; trunk control adequate for sitting; could not perform rapid, alternating movements. Skin: no lesions.

Laboratory Findings: *On admission*—EEG: positive (background asymmetry and multifocal sharp waves not associated with clinical seizures). CSF: WBCs present. CT and MRI scans of head: normal. *Nine days later*—Routine labs, including electrolytes, BUN, creatinine, thyroid studies, liver functions: normal. Amylase, lipase, folate, albumin, vitamin B-12: normal. CSF: clear with < 10 mg/dl protein, glucose 48, and 0-1 RBCs, 137 WBC, 1% neutrophils, 82% lymphocytes, 9% monocytes, and 1% basophils. Cultures and studies for infectious agents, including cryptococcal antigen: negative. Detailed study of CSF proteins, including immunoglobulins: unrevealing, except IgG to albumin ratio mildly elevated at 0.24 (top normal 0.21); only one oligoclonal band. Urinalysis: normal. Serum IGA 255, C3 139, C4 26.9. HIV ab: negative. CD3, CD4, CD8, CD19: normal. Monotest and CRP screen: negative.

Rocky Mountain spotted fever and related latex agglutinations: negative. TB skin test: negative. Meningoencephalitis panel: Epstein Barr virus–associated nuclear antigen 1:80, indicating past EBV infection; "mid-range positive" Mycoplasma titer, also indicating past infection. No evidence for herpesvirus, enterovirus, or the suspected arbovirus infection. Drug screens (for amphetamine and barbiturate): negative. CBC: WBC 13,500/µl, HGB/HCT 14.1/42.0, normal red cell indices, differential 3% monocytes, 25% lymphocytes, 56% neutrophils, 13% bands, 2% myelocytes, 1% variant lymphocytes; platelets 329,000/µl. Direct and indirect Coombs' tests: negative. ANA titer: 1:20, with speckled pattern. Lupus anticoagulant and anticardiolipins: negative. Nuclear antigen with and without RNase, RNP, anti-Smith, ENA, anti-DNA, and PM-1: negative.

Question: She is not getting any better; in fact she gradually becomes dependent for all activities of daily living, including mobility. What other diagnosis should be entertained?

Diagnosis: Lupus cerebritis

Discussion: Initially, the cause of this patient's disorder was considered to be an unknown infectious agent with functional overlay. The positive ANA titer seemed highly suggestive, but the rheumatology consultant believed that this was just another red herring, as false positives are common in the setting of infectious disease. The lab findings indicated no active infection.

Though a psychiatric or nonorganic etiology such as hysterical psychosis and gait disorder was considered as well, continued observation made it clear that the patient really had ataxia, not astasia-abasia. She became even less coherent, often with anxious affect and agitation. Brain SPECT 5 days after she was accepted for rehabilitation showed decreased perfusion in the right temporal lobe

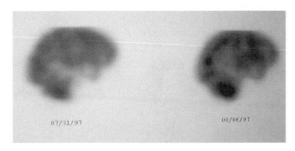

extending minimally into the right parietal lobe (see figure). No other abnormalities were found.

The psychiatry resident who consulted on the case was puzzled because so many features did not fit a diagnosis of first schizophrenic break: the patient went from well-adjusted to physically incapacitated (not just mentally out-of-sync with reality); a transient red malar rash in a butterfly pattern appeared at different times; the ANA persisted, with a titer as high as 1:80; and a repeat anti-DNA was weakly positive. Although some consultants were skeptical, a literature review suggested that this is not an unheard-of presentation for lupus cerebritis; after some argument she was started on IV methylprednisolone, and then switched to oral steroids when she started to improve dramatically.

Follow-up SPECT studies at 1 and 2 weeks showed continued improvement in blood flow to the right temporal lobe. Eventually, this flow normalized; increased blood flow in the left basal ganglia and thalamus also normalized on the final study. Repeat CSF studies were normal. She eventually returned to finish high school successfully. She has some steroid side effects, but no other deficits cognitively or physically.

Clinical Pearls

1. Systemic lupus erthyematosus can present as an isolated cerebritis, looking for all the world like an organic psychosis, and is highly treatable.

2. SPECT scan can show abnormalities of function in the absence of structural findings.

3. Infectious causes that don't get better and show no white matter or immunologic changes, or psychiatric disorders that don't fit any DSM-III or IV criteria for anything common to the age group, may be something else entirely.

4. When a good program of rehabilitation therapy fails to show expected improvement in function, strongly consider medical illness as the underlying problem.

REFERENCES

1. Asherson RA, Denburg SD, Denburg JA, et al: Current concepts of neuropsychiatric systemic lupus erythematosus (NP-SLE). Postgrad Med J 69(814):602–608, 1993.
2. Feinglass EJ, Arnett FC, Dorsch CA, et al: Neuropsychiatric manifestations of systemic lupus erythematosus: Diagnosis, clinical spectrum, and relationship to other features of the disease. Medicine (Baltimore) 55(4):323–339, 1976.
3. Kohen M, Asherson RA, Gharavi AE, Lahita RG: Lupus psychosis: Differentiation from the steroid-induced state. Clin Exp Rheumatol 11(3):323–326, 1993.
4. Sherer Y, Levy Y, Langevitz P, et al: Successful treatment of systemic lupus erythematosus cerebritis with intravenous immunoglobulin. Clin Rheumatol 18(2):170–173, 1999.
5. West SG: Neuropsychiatric lupus. Rheum Dis Clin North Am 20(1):129-158, 1994.

PATIENT 82

A 48-year-old man with paraplegia and a swollen left leg

A 48-year-old, obese man with paraplegia secondary to a logging accident presents to your clinic complaining of left leg swelling which has grown worse over the last week. He has a complete spinal cord injury, but complains that something just does not feel right. He completed a 12-week course of anticoagulation during his acute rehabilitation stay on the spinal cord injury service under your care. He has been home for 1 month and denies any falls or trauma to the left leg. He reports no fever or chills and otherwise feels good. The swelling in his left leg has appeared slowly and is getting worse, and he is having trouble getting a shoe on the left foot.

Physical Examination: Temperature 98.2°; pulse 92; respirations 18; blood pressure 102/60. HEENT: normal. Chest: clear. Cardiac: normal. Abdomen: nontender, with normal active bowel sounds. Musculoskeletal: bilateral leg swelling, but much worse on left compared to right. Extremities: 3+ edema of left leg and calf, 1+ edema of right leg and calf; full range of motion of bilateral legs, but with minimal loss of range with left hip external rotation. Skin: no skin breakdown on either leg, over the sacrum, or in ischial areas; no warmth or skin color changes.

Laboratory Findings: WBC 8500/µl; hct 32.4%; platelets 155,000/µl. Urinalysis: occasional WBCs, large amount of bacteria, leukocyte esterase negative, nitrate negative. BUN 21 mg/dl, creatinine 1.1 mg/dl, albumin 4 g/dl. Doppler ultrasound of bilateral legs: normal for deep venous system. Bone scan: see figure.

Question: What is the diagnosis?

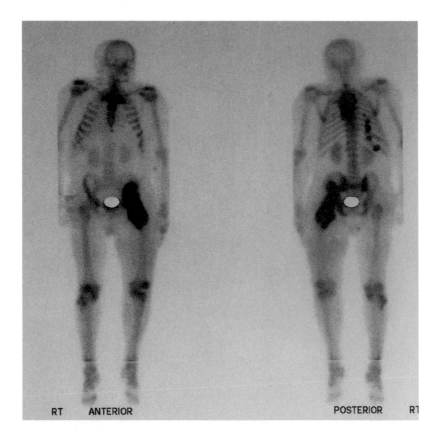

RT   ANTERIOR   POSTERIOR   RT

Diagnosis: Left hip heterotopic ossification.

Discussion: Heterotopic ossification (HO) is the development of bone in periarticular soft tissue. It was first described in spinal cord injury in 1918. The incidence of HO in patients with spinal cord injury is 10–52%. The incidence of bony ankylosis in individuals with HO is 5%, and approximately 20% of patients will have some functional loss of range of motion. The etiology of HO is unknown, but the proposed mechanism suggests the differentiation of pluripotent mesenchymal cells to osteoblastic stem cells in the post-traumatic period.

Dependent edema is quite common in spinal cord injury, especially in a patient who is sitting up more in a wheelchair. A deep vein thrombosis (DVT) and/or fracture is high on the differential diagnosis list. HO can mimic a DVT because the early clinical signs are swelling and warmth. A concurrent ipsilateral DVT can develop along with active HO.

The prognosis is greatly improved if the HO is diagnosed early and an aggressive range-of-motion program is started. Disodium etidronate has been shown to effectively limit the extent of ossification if started early. A dose of 20 mg/kg of disodium etidronate is given for 2 weeks, followed by 10 mg/kg for 10 weeks. Garland et al. suggest that 20 mg/kg for 6 months after early diagnosis would be more effective.

If anklyosis and loss of function occur, however, the only effective treatment to restore functional range of motion is surgical resection of the HO. Surgery is usually combined with radiation therapy and disodium etidronate or an NSAID, or both, because of the recurrence of HO after surgery. The timing of surgery is debated, but is usually scheduled after the HO is determined to be mature based on follow-up bone scans. Maturity is usually reached 12–18 months after the initial clinical presentation. However, Freebourn et al. reported one case in which immature HO by bone scan was resected successfully only 11 months after the initial presentation. Postoperatively, the patient received 700 cGy of radiation and indomethacin 25 mg tid for 6 weeks. His range of motion for hip flexion improved from 75 degrees preoperatively to 110 degrees postoperatively.

The present patient reported leg swelling of 1-week duration and no history of trauma to the leg. However, with a normal Doppler ultrasound and no other explanation, HO must be considered. As can be seen in the bone scan, a significant amount of bone formation is occurring around the left hip. He was started on indomethacin and disodium etidronate. Unfortunately, when attempting to transfer and lift his leg up onto the exercise mat in the physical therapy gym, he sustained a proximal femur fracture of the left lower extremity. Because of the location of the fracture, open reduction and fixation with an intramedullary nail were required. Despite treatment with etidronate, indomethacin, and range-of-motion exercises, he lost approximately 20 degrees of hip flexion. This was accommodated in his wheel chair with an increased back angle and a gel wheelchair cushion, with trimming of the solid foam cushion to allow increased hip extension when sitting. He did not require surgical resection of the heterotopic bone.

Clinical Pearls

1. Heterotopic ossification (HO) in spinal cord injury can clinically mimic a deep vein thrombosis (DVT) and occur at the same time as a DVT.

2. Prognosis is greatly improved if diagnosed early and aggressively treated with range of motion, disodium etidronate, and/or an NSAID.

3. Once HO is diagnosed, 5% of patients go on to have bony ankylosis and 20% have some functional loss.

4. Surgical resection is the only treatment option to improve range of motion, once the joint has lost range. The timing of surgery is usually after the HO is mature on bone scan, but this is under debate.

5. HO will recur after surgical resection; therefore, radiation, a disphosphonate, and/or an NSAID are recommended postoperatively.

REFERENCES

1. Bradleigh LH, Perkash A, Linder SH, et al: Deep venous thrombosis associated with heterotopic ossification. Arch Phys Med Rehabil 73:293–294,1992.
2. Freebourn TM, Barber DB, Able AC: The treatment of immature heterotopic ossification in spinal cord injury with combination surgery, radiation therapy, and NSAID. Spinal Cord 37:50–53,1999.
3. Garland DE, Alday B, Venos KG, Vogt JC: Disphosphonate treatment for heterotopic ossification in spinal cord injury patients. Clin Ortho Rel Res 176:197–200, 1983.
4. Singer BR: Heterotopic ossification. Br J Hosp Med 49:247–255, 1993.
5. Staas WE Jr, Formal CS, Gershkoff AM, et al: Rehabilitation of the spinal cord–injured patient. In Delisa JA (ed): Rehabilitation Medicine: Principles and Practice. Philadelphia, JB Lippincott Co., 1993, pp 894–895.

PATIENT 83

**A 28-year-old woman with an above-knee amputation
and prosthetic knee buckling**

A 28-year-old woman had a mid-thigh transfemoral (above-knee) amputation 10 months ago due to trauma from a motor vehicular accident. She is an executive secretary and generally wears high-heels at work. She has been wearing her definitive prosthesis for the last 5 months. This prosthesis has a total contact ischial containment suction socket with a thermoflex liner, a swing and stance phase-control hydraulic knee, and an energy-storing Carbon Copy II foot. After some minor adjustments, she has not had any problems until recently, when she noticed a tendency for the prosthetic knee to buckle at heel strike. Review of systems is negative for any recent body weight changes.

Physical Examination: General: alert and oriented times three, well developed, no acute distress. Musculoskeletal: strength 5/5 in upper and lower extremities, including hip and residual limb muscles. Gait: buckling of prosthetic knee at heel strike—approximately 50% of the time with shoes; almost none of the time without shoes.

Question: What is the cause of this amputee's gait abnormality?

Answer: Shoe heel height incompatible with prosthetic alignment

Discussion: Buckling of the knee during heel strike in a transfemoral amputee's prosthesis can be due to the following:

- Excessive dorsiflexion of the foot
- Improper knee joint alignment (knee center is forward relative to weight line)
- Weakness of the gluteus maximus
- Lack of friction in the knee joint mechanism
- Change in shoe heel height, to one higher than that originally used for alignment.

The present patient showed more knee stability when she walked without her shoes, indicating that the cause of the prosthetic knee buckling was due to a higher heel. Hence, the solution was to wear shoes with heels that have the same height as the ones originally used when alignment of her prosthesis was done.

Clinical Pearls

1. Evaluate the gait of lower extremity amputees both with and without their shoes.
2. Examine the strength of the hip girdle, as well as the more distal muscles of the residual limb.

REFERENCES

1. Berger N: Gait deviations and lower-limb prostheses. In O'Young B, Young MA, Stiens SA (eds): PM&R Secrets. Philadelphia, Hanley & Belfus, 1997, pp 565–569.
2. Friedman LW: Rehabilitation of the lower extremity amputee. In Kottke FJ, Lehmann JF (eds): Krusen's Handbook of Physical Medicine and Rehabilitation, 4th ed. Philadelphia, WB Saunders, 1990, pp 1024–1069.
3. Leonard JA, Meier RH: Upper and lower extremity prosthetics. In Delisa JA, Gans BM (eds): Rehabilitation Medicine: Principles and Practice, 3rd ed. Philadelphia, Lippincott-Raven, 1998, pp 669–696.

PATIENT 84

A 20-year-old man with tetraplegia and hemoptysis

A 20-year-old man was injured in a motor vehicle accident 3 weeks ago when the car he was riding in was struck by an 18-wheel truck. He sustained a C5 fracture and underwent anterior cervical discectomy and fusion. He is now on the spinal cord injury ward at the rehabilitation hospital. He is classified as a C6 incomplete spinal cord injury, American Spinal Injury Association impairment scale B. You are called by the house physician in the evening because the patient is anxious and complaining of a headache, as well as chest pain and shortness of breath. His blood pressure is 162/65, and he is running a fever of 102.4° F. His bladder was just catheterized and revealed only 250 cc of cloudy urine. The bowel program has not been completed yet because the patient's family is visiting, and he requested a delay.

Physical Examination: *That evening*—Temperature 102.4°; pulse 92; respirations 18; blood pressure 162/60. HEENT: face flushed and sweating; pupils equal, round, and react to light and accomodation; extraocular muscles intact. Chest: clear. Cardiac: normal. Abdomen: nontender, with normal active bowel sounds. Musculoskeletal: no lower extremity swelling or redness. Skin: stage 2 sacral pressure ulcer, unchanged from earlier in the week, and no signs of infection; no other signs of pressure sores or skin irritation.

The bowel program is completed satisfactorily 2 hours later, with no evidence of impaction, and the patient begins to rest more comfortably. His blood pressure decreases to 120/55 and pulse to 80. He is still somewhat anxious, but sleeps through the night.

Next morning—General: slightly anxious. Blood pressure: 100/50. Because he was feeling ill, physical therapy was conducted bedside. However, he had a sudden episode of coughing and hemoptysis.

Laboratory Findings: WBC 8700/μl; hct 32.4%; platelets 155,000/μl. Troponin 1 < 0.1, CPK 960. Urinalysis: 2–5 WBCs, large amount of bacteria, leukocyte esterase positive, nitrate negative. BUN: 21 mg/dl, creatinine 0.9 mg/dl, albumin 4 g/dl. Pulse oximetry (room air): 99%. Doppler ultrasound of bilateral legs: normal for deep venous system. Chest x-ray: normal. V/Q scan: see figure.

Question: What is the diagnosis?

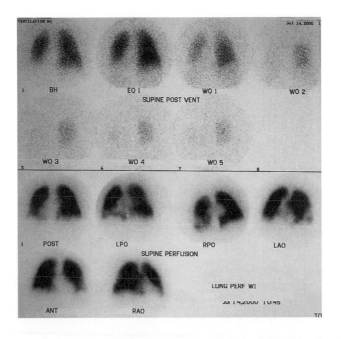

Diagnosis: Autonomic dysreflexia secondary to a pulmonary embolus.

Discussion: The most frequent signs and symptoms of autonomic dysreflexia are paroxysmal hypertension causing pounding headaches, visual disturbance, and/or chest pain. Additional features are sympathetic inhibitory outflow resulting in sweating, and vasodilatation resulting in skin flushing. Autonomic dysreflexia can occur after the phase of spinal shock has resolved and the patient's reflexes are returning. If the SCI is above the major splanchnic outflow (T6–L2), the potential is high for developing this disorder.

Autonomic dysreflexia results from various noxious stimuli, which in turn trigger sympathetic hyperactivity. The list of causes of noxious stimuli in an individual with SCI is long and wide-ranging. Stimulation from the lower urinary tract accounts for the majority of episodes, with bladder distention accounting for 75–85% of these. The second most common cause is anorectal stimulation with bowel distention due to fecal impaction, which accounts for 13–19% of occurrences. After these two, any noxious stimuli you can think of can result in autonomic dysreflexia in SCI with a level of approximately T6 or higher. Note that pulmonary embolus is a recognized cause of autonomic dysreflexia.

The risk of thromboembolism after an SCI is high and increases rapidly after an injury, reaching a maximal risk 7–10 days after the acute injury. Incidence is low during the first 72 hours, but starting heparin within 72 hours of the SCI is recommended. The incidence of thromboembolism with the use of low-dose heparin is 7–50%, and with the use of low-molecular-weight heparin, 0–8%. In a patient with autonomic dysreflexia, if the symptoms do not resolve with the proper management of bowel and bladder, then medication should be used to lower the blood pressure until the source of the noxious stimulation is found. Nifedipine is a good choice as it is a short-acting antihypertensive medication that has been used safely for years. Another good choice is nitropaste, which can be removed once the noxious stimulation is found. However, if nitropaste is to be used you must ensure that the patient is not taking sildenafil (Viagra) for erectile dysfunction, as the two can cause acute and life-threatening hypotension.

The present patient had some of the common symptoms of autonomic dysreflexia, and the appropriate measures were taken to manage bowel and bladder—with some success. However, he was still apprehensive and not feeling well the next morning. The patient had been on appropriate prophylaxis for deep vein thrombosis (DVT) with sequential compression hose in the hospital, and transition to low-molecular-weight heparin occurred 72 hours after the injury. He was on gastrointestinal prophylaxis with an H2 blocker. The sudden episode of hematemesis may have been the result of a gastrointestinal bleed or an acute pulmonary embolus. On assessment of the hematemesis you note a large blood clot, but no other fluid, which leads you to suspect an acute pulmonary embolus and order a ventilation/perfusion (V/Q) scan and a Doppler ultrasound to assess for a DVT in both legs. The V/Q scan (see figure) is consistent with a high-probability pulmonary embolus, and the patient is transferred to the medical intensive care unit for acute management.

Clinical Pearls

1. Autonomic dysreflexia in spinal cord injury (SCI) occurs when the level of the SCI is above the major splanchnic outflow (T6–L2), and is the result of a noxious stimulation below the level of the SCI.

2. The major sources of noxious stimulation that result in autonomic dysreflexia in SCI are bladder (75–85%) and bowel (13–19%).

3. If the source of the noxious stimulation cannot be located after bowel and bladder management and a quick skin examination, treat the blood pressure with medication, and investigate other sources of noxious stimulation.

4. If a patient is on sildenafil (Viagra) for erectile dysfunction, do not use any products with nitrates to lower the blood pressure, as there is a risk of life-threatening hypotension.

REFERENCES

1. Apple DF: Autonomic dysreflexia management. American Spinal Injury Association newsletter 1999.
2. Cheitlin MD, et al: Use of sildenafil (Viagra) in patients with cardiovascular disease. Circulation 99:168–177, 1999.
3. Colachis SC III: Autonomic hyperreflexia in spinal cord injury associated with pulmonary embolism. Arch Phys Med Rehabil 72:1014–1016, 1991.
4. Consortium for Spinal Cord Medicine: Acute Management of Autonomic Dysreflexia: Adults with Spinal Cord Injury Presenting to Healthcare Facilities. Washington DC, Paralyzed Veterans of America, February 1997.
5. Consortium for Spinal Cord Medicine: Prevention of Thromboembolism in Spinal Cord Injury. Washington DC, Paralyzed Veterans of America, February 1997.
6. Lee BY, Karmakar MG, Herz BL, Sturgill RA: Autonomic dysreflexia revisited. J Spinal Cord Med 18:75–87,1995.

PATIENT 85

A 2-year-old boy with unexplained motor findings

A 2-year-old boy is referred because he just started walking at 20 months and his feet are turning in. He started cruising at 17 months. He was born at term weighing 7 lbs 7 oz, with no complications. He has no prior illness and no family history of developmental disorders. There is no history of loss or regression of milestones.

Physical Examination: Weight 14.5 kg, height 88 cm, head circumference 49.7 cm. General: he likes to W-sit and shows some femoral anteversion and internal tibial torsion. Neurologic: deep tendon reflexes brisk; mild clonus at ankles; Babinski reflexes equivocal; tone normal to mildly increased distally in lower extremities. Musculoskeletal: gait wide-based; tends toward mild excess plantarflexion dynamically; passive range of motion full throughout.

Laboratory Findings: CT scan of head: cerebellar atrophy. Serum and urine amino acid screens: normal. Creatinine phosphokinase: 68.

Question: The mother was told after this initial examination that her son had very mild ataxic cerebral palsy, needing only a home program with limited outpatient therapy. What else should have been considered?

Answer: Neurodegenerative diseases, specifically leukodystrophy

Discussion: An orthopedist who sees the patient 16 months later notes that he falls more frequently and has enough dynamic equinus to warrant use of inhibitive ankle-foot orthoses. He returns at 3 years of age to the pediatric physiatrist with clearly more increased tone, some right upper extremity tightness, and gross truncal ataxia. An MRI scan shows not just cerebellar atrophy, but also **absent myelination** (see figure). He is seen in a neurogenetics clinic, where his very long-chain fatty acids are found to be elevated. Fibroblast culture from skin biopsy confirms a diagnosis of **metachromatic leukodystrophy**.

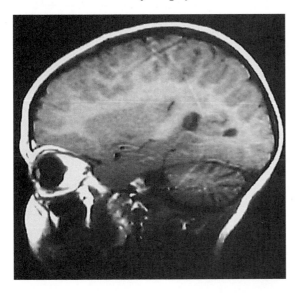

The patient continues to receive follow-up in an habilitation clinic, no longer walking even in therapy by age 8.5, needing full trunk support in sitting by age 10.5, and showing early signs of dysphagia and loss of head control when fatigued at age 13. Cognitive and behavioral limitations became evident in early school years. He attends special camp every summer and uses a computer for some play and communication activities.

Although in years past it was taught that most cerebral palsy is idiopathic, this may no longer be true and, in fact, gives a false sense of security. This child's mother first had to adjust to her child's diagnosis of cerebral palsy (static encephalopathy), which she did admirably; the readjustment to the diagnosis of a progressive and eventually life-limiting disease was much more emotionally difficult. This scenario is not uncommon among parents of children with neurodegenerative disease. They often speak wistfully of the days "when we thought he just had cerebral palsy."

No disease-modifying treatment was available to help this young man, but experimental therapies such as bone marrow transplantation are becoming available, making early diagnosis even more critical. What was done correctly in this case was to plan follow-up visits, recognize changes beyond the usual evolution of abnormal tone (children with cerebral palsy may show increases in spasticity and movement disorders in their first few years), and reassess the diagnosis. Getting a creatinine phosphokinase level was not unreasonable, as some children with Duchenne's dystrophy present as mildly delayed with mildly abnormal tone, though they do not have true ataxia or hyperreflexia, and would not be toe-walking so early in most cases. Amino acid screening and thyroid testing completed the traditional trio of basic lab work for unexplained developmental delay, though those metabolic disorders usually affect cognitive development earlier and to a greater extent than motor. Thyroid testing was omitted because growth was normal, and there were no symptoms or signs to suggest hypothyroidism. Moreover, he had usual screening at birth since his was a hospital delivery.

Purely ataxic cerebral palsy due to a static cerebellar abnormality does exist, but leukodystrophy or metabolic disorder such as carbohydrate-deficient glycoprotein syndrome should be considered. Dandy Walker cysts or other posterior fossa anomaly would be better assessed by MRI than CT also. "Bulbar cerebral palsy," which combines mild ataxia and spasticity with some involvement of speech and swallowing, is most usually due to periventricular leukomalacia more posteriorly in the cerebral hemispheres. In this case there was no prematurity to predispose to intraventricular hemorrhage or perinatal stressor, which can rarely cause this in a term infant.

Clinical Pearls

1. "Cerebral palsy" in a term baby with no explanation needs to be further evaluated.
2. "Ataxic cerebral palsy" does exist, but deserves a more detailed workup.
3. Children may initially make progress outstripping that of a progressive neurodegenerative disease; the innate drive towards normal development and function is a powerful force.
4. MRI is the neuroimaging study of choice to assess white matter disease.

REFERENCES

1. Aicardi J: The inherited leukodystrophies: a clinical overview. J Inherit Metab Dis 16(4):733–743, 1993.
2. Kolodny EH: Dysmyelinating and demyelinating conditions in infancy. Curr Opin Neurol Neurosurg 6(3):379–386, 1993.
3. Powers JM, Rubio A: Selected leukodystrophies. Semin Pediatr Neurol 2(3):200–210, 1995.

INDEX